CONSTIPATION, PILES AND OTHER BOWEL DISORDERS

OTHER BOOKS IN THE SERIES

IN PREPARATION

CONSTIPATION, PILES AND OTHER BOWEL DISORDERS

RICHARD HEATLEY MD, MRCP
Senior Lecturer in Medicine,
University of Leeds, and
Consultant Physician
St James University Hospital, Leeds

Foreword by
Dr Denis Burkitt

Cartoons by *David Nathanson*

Churchill Livingstone

EDINBURGH LONDON MELBOURNE AND NEW YORK 1984

CHURCHILL LIVINGSTONE
Medical Division of Longman Group Limited

Distributed in the United States of America by Churchill
Livingstone Inc., 1560 Broadway, New York, N.Y. 10036,
and by associated companies, branches and representatives
throughout the world.

First published 1984

ISBN 0 443 02915 6

British Library Cataloguing in Publication Data

Heatley, R. V.
    Constipation, piles and other bowel disorders. —
    (Patient handbooks ; no. 17)
    1. Constipation.
    I. Title   II. Series
    616.3'42   RC861

Library of Congress Cataloging in Publication Data

Heatley, Richard.
    Constipation, piles and other bowel disorders.
    (Patient handbooks ; 17)
    1. Intestines — Diseases. 2. Constipation. 3. Hemorrhoids.
I. Title II. Series: Churchill Livingstone patient handbook ;
17. [DNLM: 1. Intestinal diseases — Popular works.
2. Constipation — Popular works. 3. Hemorrhoids —
Popular works. WI 400 H441c]
RC860.H43   1984   616.3'4   83-20905

Printed in Singapore by
The Print House Pte Ltd

FOREWORD

Regrettably the subject of bowel behaviour is in many cultures, including modern Western society, a taboo subject. It is considered extremely personal yet to each individual it is of profound importance. The very fact that there is reluctance to discuss the matter makes it particularly necessary that suitable literature should be available that supplies reliable information in an understandable form.

This book by Dr R V Heatley does just that. It sets out in simple language the functions of the different parts of the digestive tract, explains what may go wrong and how the resultant ailments can best be managed. It dispels time-honoured but fanciful myths, justly warns against injudicious use of laxatives and refutes the common notion that diarrhoea demands immediate medication.

There is sound guidance on when and when not to bother your doctor, and since food is naturally of great importance in the causation, prevention and treatment of bowel disorders there are helpful, practical and sound guide-lines with regard to a healthy diet. The knowledge contained in this excellent and highly commendable book will do much to allay anxieties, prevent disease, and enable readers to deal with their own bowel problems when mild, and direct them to their doctor when professional advice is required.

1984   Denis Burkitt

DR DENIS BURKITT
CMG MD DSc FRCS FRCPI FRS

Dr Burkitt is among the world's leading pioneers in demonstrating the benefits of dietary fibre. Having worked for many years in Africa, he was one of those who drew attention to the possible effects of our ever changing diet in causing many of the common diseases in the Western world. His undaunted efforts over the years have helped to make fibre a household word in this country and have done much to make people aware of the importance of diet in preserving good health.

CONTENTS

1. WHAT MAKES MY BOWELS GO WRONG?

Is this a book for me?

The problems caused by bowel disorders are familiar to more of us than are likely to admit it. Constipation, diarrhoea, abdominal cramps and wind are symptoms we have probably all experienced at one time or another. And yet, digestive disorders, widespread as they are, rarely get talked about. Although we regard ourselves as being enlightened about health matters compared with our predecessors, many freely talk about health risks affecting the reproductive system and sexual function but behave as if our bowels do not exist. The amount of distress and embarrassment digestive upsets cause to millions of people vastly exceeds the frequency with which they are discussed among friends and acquaintances. Because they are so little talked about and so poorly understood, many people suffer needlessly for years, often compounding their problem by their concern and the remedies they themselves choose. Sometimes the symptoms signal a serious underlying disease that, if neglected, can cause irrevocable damage and even death. Other times the symptoms merely mimic those of serious disorders and cause more emotional distress than the actual physical situation warrants. More often than not, however, prompt and accurate diagnosis and proper treatment can greatly reduce the mental and physical stress and halt or even reverse the underlying disorder. For instance, cancer of the bowels, a subject you hardly ever hear about, kills over 16 000 people each year in England and Wales alone, more than die from breast cancer and it is one of the forms of cancer which is curable if detected early enough. At present though, only about 1 in 10 cases is discovered at an early stage. Furthermore, those who do suffer with digestive diseases must cope not only with what can be debilitating, long-standing disorders but also with the general public's aversion to open discussions of bowel function. Even reporting the reasons for absence from work or social activities because of bowel disorders can be embarrassing for many. And yet, digestive disorders are widespread. Each year in this country, family doctors are consulted on over 4 million occasions (this involves around 1 in every 6 of these doctors' patients) because of digestive upsets and about half a million people are referred to hospital each year for these problems.

What are my bowels and what do they do?

The bowels are the small and large intestines. These are part of the digestive system which is a long hollow tube very similar to a hose-pipe beginning at the lips and mouth and running through the body to end at the back passage (the rectum and anus).

The small intestine is about 20 feet long and lies coiled in the central part of the tummy (abdomen) around the region of the navel (umbilicus). Digestive secretions are emptied into the intestine from glands, the liver and pancreas and food and drink is digested inside the hollow intestine. The resulting chemicals filter across the intestinal lining into the bloodstream and then pass to the liver to be re-formed into other chemicals which then travel off in the bloodstream again to build new tissues elsewhere in the body. The upper

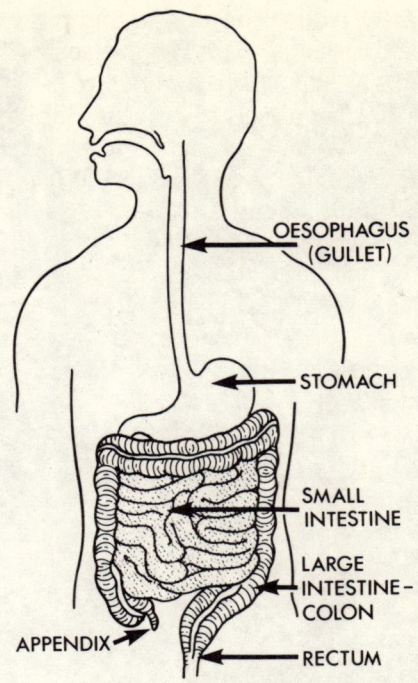

Fig. 1 A diagram of the digestive system

part of the small intestine is known as the jejunum, the remaining lower portion the ileum.

The first part of the large intestine leading on from the terminal ileum (the end portion of the small intestine) is a large expandable sack, the caecum, from which the appendix comes off. The appendix is a small, blind-ending tube with no known function. The remainder of the large intestine is the colon (which is about 5 feet long) and lies around the outer margin of the abdominal cavity and ends in the back passage (the rectum); the opening to the exterior being the anus, through which waste material in the form of faeces is evacuated.

After digestion is completed and the useful constituents of the diet are removed, some undigestible and indestruct-

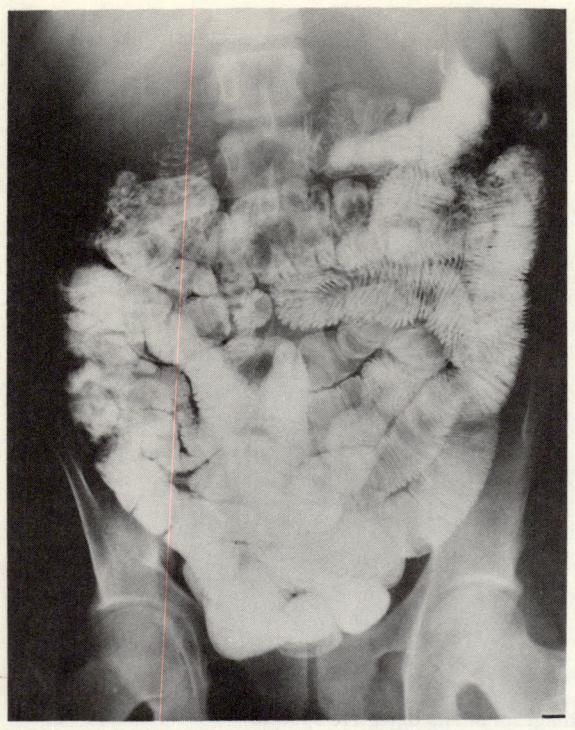

Fig. 2 A barium X-ray showing the small intestine. Each loop of bowel shows up in white and has a 'striped' appearance because of folds in the intestine — it is like a concertina.

ible components of food remain lying inside the hollow small intestine. Continuous muscular contractions force this onward into the large intestine. However, the body has not yet finished with it, although most is waste. The large intestine concentrates the waste from the digestive processes by continuing muscular contraction to compress it and water and salts are removed from the contents and reabsorbed into the body to be conserved.

The colon acts as a reservoir for waste material where it is

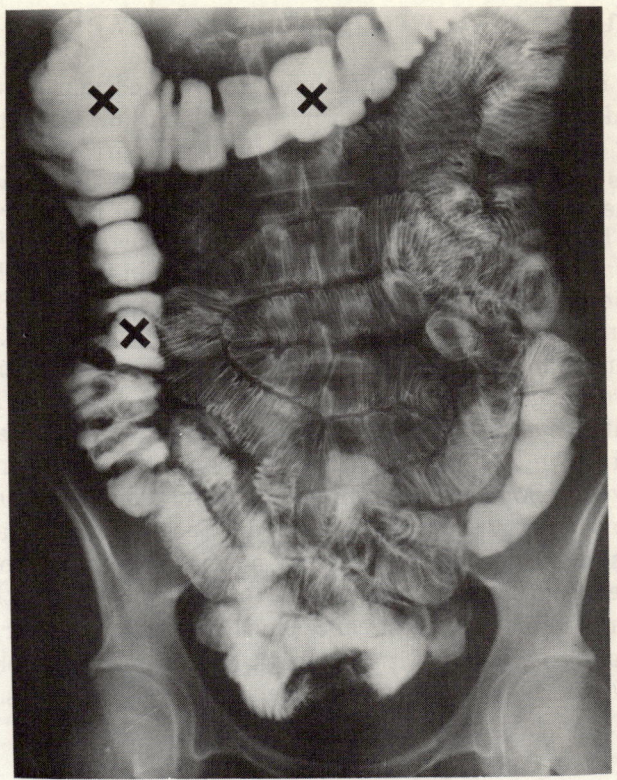

Fig. 3 A barium X-ray, showing in the centre the small intestine and around the outside the large intestine (colon) which is marked X.

temporarily stored. Periodical muscular contractions slowly move the contents through the colon. Stronger, more wide-spread, co-ordinated, muscular action often stimulated by the volume of faecal material, movement of the body (taking exercise) or filling of the stomach by a further meal, cause evacuation of the contents. The muscles around the back passage open to allow the contents of the bowel to leave but shut tightly again afterwards to prevent leakage.

What can go wrong with the bowels?

The intestines are part of a long, hollow muscular tube supplied by blood vessels and nerves, which link them to the rest of the body. Diseases can affect any part of the intestines and, by means of these connections, the body as a whole. Generalised diseases of the body can cause bowel trouble and bowel diseases can also affect other parts of the body.

Many types of different problems occur in the bowels. Infections passed on by eating or drinking contaminated food or drink or contact with other people suffering from gastroenteritis are common problems especially for people travelling abroad and also for children. There are also some types of intestinal inflammation which occur for reasons that are not fully understood and can cause bowel trouble on and off for years. Some of the commonest bowel troubles occurring in this country are thought to be due to the poorly balanced diets we eat which disturb the normal movements of the bowel. Cancer can also affect the intestines and since this is a fairly common type of cancer in this country it is very important to recognise it early as it can often be completely cured and is probably also preventable in many cases.

What causes gastroenteritis?

A large number of infections caused by bacteria, viruses or parasites (worms) can affect the intestines to cause gastroenteritis. Although the stomach is often involved early as well, so that vomiting results, the more striking and longlasting effects are most commonly related to the intestines. Most infections are caused by taking contaminated food or water, although some of the viruses may be passed on by inhalation. In this country water from cold taps (i.e. straight from the mains supply) is invariably safe, but this is not necessarily the case in other parts of the world. Contamination of food or drink by contact with human excrement because of poor personal hygiene is one of the commonest means of transmission. Organisms themselves need not necessarily enter the body to cause illness. Bacteria multiplying on food produce toxins (poisons), which cause symptoms when eaten. The commonest causes for this are inadequately re-heated food or cream cakes which have been left uncovered and become contaminated by flies.

Gastroenteritis is commonly a mild illness, but can be severe. It often starts suddenly and is accompanied by varying degrees of vomiting, griping abdominal pain, diarrhoea and general weakness. It usually clears up by itself within a few days and almost always within a couple of weeks.

Parasitic infections of the gut are common worldwide but uncommon in Britain. Threadworm infections not uncommonly affect children and cause intense itching around the back passage. Other parasite infections can be caught by eating undercooked food, especially pork and fish, and drinking contaminated water. They can cause a variety of gut disturbances.

What causes intestinal inflammation?

Coeliac disease

This is a rare condition, caused by wheat in the diet. In this disorder, a constituent of wheat (gluten, which is the part of wheat that makes dough, doughy) damages the lining of the small intestine and this interferes with digestion. Once diagnosed, it is a life-long condition and can be controlled by totally avoiding wheat in the diet. This sounds easy, but is not always the case, since wheat in cereals, flour, and bread is a very common constituent of all of our diets, as it occurs in gravy, tinned foods, pies and pastry and many other foods. Coeliac disease is probably in part inherited since it is more common in families with affected individuals and is especially common on the West coast of Ireland. It causes anaemia, diarrhoea, abdominal distension, loss of weight and failure to grow in children, and occasionally it can cause skin rashes. It is not clear how wheat damages the bowel but it may be due to an allergic reaction. Continuation of the diet for life is vital since otherwise the condition may relapse, and cause recurrent problems and in rare instances, cancer of the intestine. Otherwise, the disease is completely controlled in the majority of patients by the total exclusion of wheat from the diet.

A very similar type of disorder, called sprue, occurs in people who have spent some time in the tropics. This is probably caused in most people by infection and can usually be cured by antibiotics — although this can sometimes be difficult to achieve.

Crohn's disease

Is called this after a Dr Crohn in New York who first discovered it in the 1930s. It causes inflammation which usually affects the small and large intestines primarily but can cause problems in any other part of the gut. The inflammation involves the gut wall and may later cause scarring and because of the swelling and damage involved can eventually encroach upon the hollow inside of the intestine and cause obstruction of the bowel or intestinal blockage. This results in abdominal cramping pains, diarrhoea, occasional vomiting, loss of weight and general ill health.

The cause is unknown, but it is believed to be due either to some sort of unusual long-standing infection or an allergic type of disorder. There is no evidence whatsoever that the disease is infective or that affected patients can pass on the disease to others, although there probably is an inherited susceptibility to it. It is becoming much more common now than it was a few years ago, particularly in the Western world.

Crohn's disease most commonly affects young people, often adolescents, but it can occur at any age. Most com-

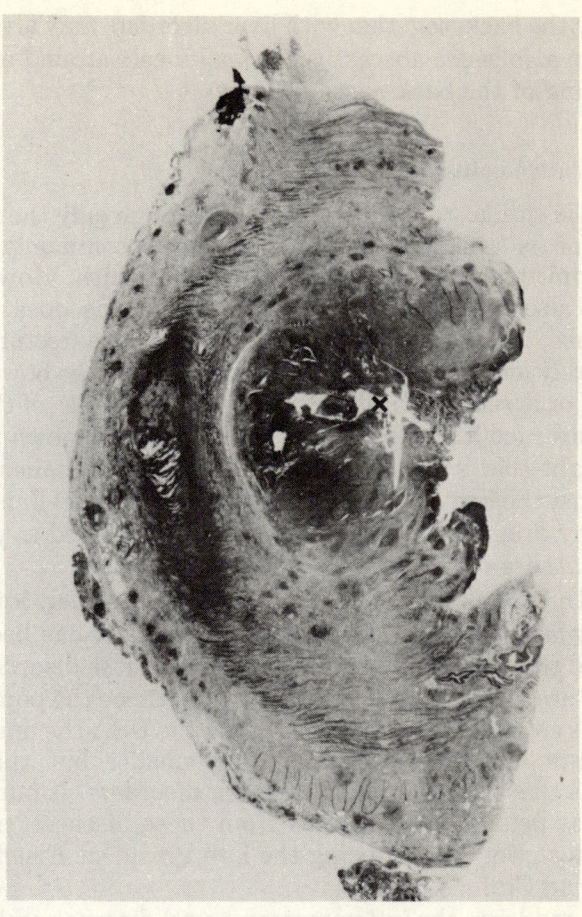

Fig. 4(a) An enlarged slice across the bowel lining in Crohn's disease. The hollow centre of the bowel (the lumen) is marked X. The intestinal wall is greatly thickened because of the inflammation and this causes narrowing of the bowel lumen which prevents food material passing through. This causes pain in the tummy and disturbance of the bowels.

monly it flares up and settles down intermittently but sometimes the symptoms are more continuous.

It is not a disease confined solely to the bowel since skin rashes, inflammation of the eyes, mouth and joints, especially the back, together with liver disorders may also occur. It can also cause abscesses or small ulcers around or at the opening of the back passage (anus).

Ulcerative colitis

This is similar to Crohn's disease although only the large intestine is affected. This disease most commonly causes intermittent bloody diarrhoea and ill health. However, it may also affect other parts of the body as does Crohn's disease. It tends to affect the back passage (rectum) most severely and may be confined to that part of the bowel (proctitis) or spread upwards to affect the remainder of the large intestine (colitis). Once again the cause is unknown but it is thought that some of the body's defence mechanisms turn against the body and start destroying the bowel lining. This is why drugs, in particular prednisone are used to dampen down these defences.

Both Crohn's disease and colitis are collectively known as *inflammatory bowel diseases*. In America it has been estimated that 2 million people suffer from these disorders and there are 100 000 new cases each year. Since the population of this country is about 1/5th that of the USA the number of patients here are proportionately smaller but that still means that they are fairly common disorders. A number of famous people have suffered from these diseases, perhaps the most well known being the late President Eisenhower, who had Crohn's disease.

By and large the inflammatory bowel diseases each cause essentially the same types of problems. On face value there is no reason why sufferers should be restricted from living an entirely normal life. However, in reality this is not so and having either Crohn's disease or colitis means in many people, interference with work and social activities even when the disease is quiescent but more so when active. Both disorders flare up unpredictably and can then cause bowel problems, both frequency and urgency of bowel actions,

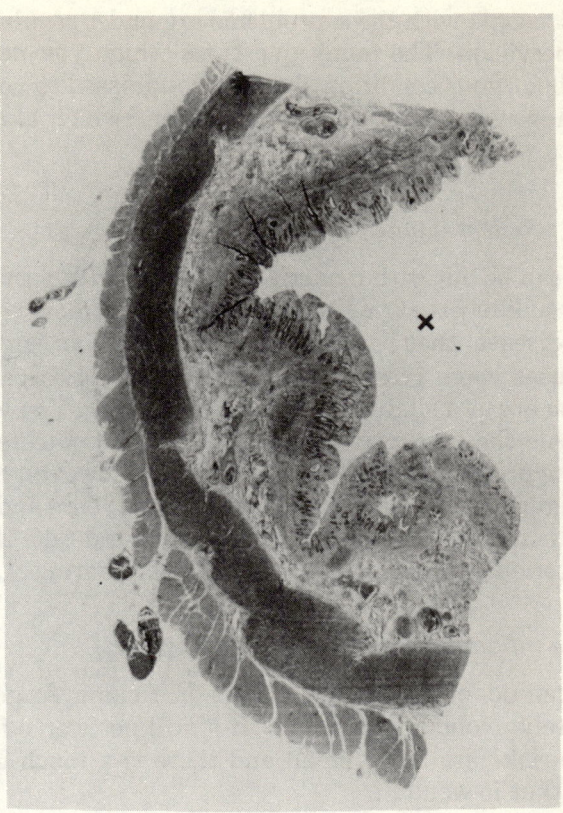

Fig. 4(b) A similar slice through the bowel in ulcerative colitis as in 4(a). Once again X marks the hollow centre of the bowel. In colitis, inflammation only affects the inner lining of the intestine and the bowel wall is no thicker than normal. Pain is therefore uncommon but bleeding from the ulcerated and inflamed lining is usual.

abdominal pain, rectal bleeding, tiredness, lassitude and weakness. Patients often fear that they will lose control of the bowels and soil their clothing or leave unpleasant smells in the toilet. On the more pleasant side there is no reason usually why pregnancy, sex or any other normal pursuit should be any different than for someone without these diseases.

Most people with these problems are under regular medical supervision. The many questions which you naturally have about your condition should be addressed to your doctors. However, there are some questions which almost all patients want answered:

Is this problem dangerous?

Yes, it can be but with modern treatment and supervision it is most unlikely that you will come to any harm. If you have severe disease, that is a lot of bowel which is inflamed and this causes you a great deal of trouble, the figures suggest that you are at a slightly greater risk of dying. You will discover this the hard way if you try and take out life insurance, the premiums will often be 'loaded'. However, most of these figures have been worked out in past years and nowadays it is unlikely, if you behave sensibly and take the condition seriously, that you will come to any harm.

Will the inflammation get worse and spread?

Yes it can do, or it can stay as it is or it can even go away completely. Nobody can predict if it will get worse for you but the risks are fairly small and there is a much greater chance that it won't.

Will I need to have an operation?

That is also, impossible to answer in any definite way. Don't forget, these tend to be lifelong conditions, there are many different reasons for advising operation (and also for *not* advising operations) and treatment is constantly changing and improving. As a general rule people with Crohn's disease are likely to need an operation of some sort sooner or later but because of the risks of later recurrence, as little will be done as needs to be. The chance of an operation for colitis is much less (if the disease is just confined to a small section of bowel, operation is most *unlikely*) but it is usually necessary to remove the whole of the large bowel if any operation is done at all.

What are the risks of getting cancer?

If you have long-standing severe ulcerative colitis which involves the whole of the colon you may eventually get cancer. This only affects a small proportion of people, however, and we are only talking about over a very long time, at least 10 if not 20 years. Nowadays these people are usually checked regularly and the bowel inspected at colonoscopy periodically. If you have less severe disease the risks of cancer are proportionately less and your doctors will advise you whether any preventative measures should be taken.

With Crohn's disease the situation is entirely different and operations to prevent cancer developing are unnecessary.

Appendicitis

The appendix is a small hollow tube about 2-4 inches long which projects from the large bowel, usually in the lower right corner of the abdomen. It does not appear to have any useful function in humans. On occasions, the internal opening of the appendix becomes blocked, although this is seldom by fruit pips or any particular constituent of the diet as was once thought. It is believed though that appendicitis occurs more commonly in people who eat a diet low in fibre. Once the blockage occurs, infection behind the blockage follows, which may spread, causing inflammation of the appendix structure itself. Unless this is treated by surgical removal, perforation of the appendix may occur which will allow infection to spread elsewhere throughout the abdomen (peritonitis). Acute appendicitis is extremely common since it affects one out of every seven people at some time in their lives. Acute appendicitis often causes initially a little crampy abdominal pain around the navel (umbilicus) or the upper part of the abdomen centrally which soon progresses to cause intense pain in the lower right portion of the abdomen. This may be accompanied by a fever, vomiting and a little diarrhoea.

What causes an irritable bowel and diverticular disease?

Irritable bowel is a condition which is also called irritable colon, irritable bowel syndrome or spastic colitis. Diverticular disease is probably also related to it.

It has become increasingly recognised in recent years that intense processing of foods to make them more palatable and easily digestible, has reduced the fibre or bulk content of our diets tremendously. This has not been the case in Africa and much of the Third World and in these countries people suffer from far less long-lasting bowel disease than in the Western world. Without bulk in the diet, the spontaneous muscular activity of the bowel is largely wasted, because there is no need to compress the waste products of digestion. As a result of this, needless high pressures are developed in the colon which can cause pain and discomfort anywhere in the abdomen due to associated bowel spasm. If this is long-standing, eventually, weaknesses (protrusions) develop in the bowel wall (diverticula). Spasm of the bowel, apart from causing abdominal pain, can lead to flatulence and bowel disturbance. This may either be constipation or increased looseness of the bowels particularly in the mornings and often urgently after meals. If this occurs, the bowel motions are fragmented and described as being like 'rabbit-droppings' or alternatively like 'toothpaste coming out of a tube'. In diverticular disease symptoms are often similar, although on occasion, the weaknesses, or little out-pouchings, which develop in the large bowel wall may become blocked off and infected. As a result areas of inflammation, perforation and occasionally peritonitis (like a 'mini'-appendicitis) can develop, which may cause severe abdominal pain (particularly on the left lower side of the abdomen), bowel disturbance and fever (acute diverticular disease or diverticulitis).

These so-called 'functional bowel disturbances' are extremely common and diverticula are present in about one-third of all people over the age of 60, although they do not necessarily cause symptoms. Although an irritable bowel and diverticular disease can cause fairly dramatic problems, sometimes severe pain and marked bowel disturbances, these conditions are not associated with any disease of the colon and except in diverticular disease the colon is not physically damaged. There is no association whatsoever between these disorders and cancer, although it is often

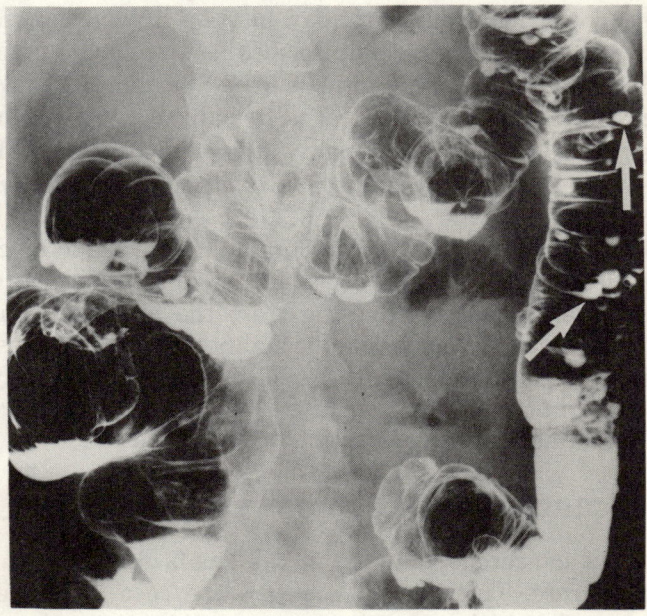

Fig. 5 A barium enema X-ray of the large intestine. Little 'outpouchings' have developed in the bowel wall (diverticula) and are shown by the arrows.

important for sufferers to be investigated to exclude cancer and other bowel disorders, since symptoms may sometimes be similar.

Can you be allergic to certain foods?

Probably, although not a great deal is known about food allergy at the present time. However, undoubtedly allergy to some food occurs in a number of bowel disorders. Some people find that they develop a skin rash after eating certain foods such as shell fish or strawberries and it is obvious that allergy is involved. However, many others suffer from more subtle disorders due to food allergy and may not have incriminated foods as precipitating agents. Food allergy has been implicated in the development of some of the functional bowel disturbances affecting the gut (such as the irritable bowel syndrome). It may also be involved in some patients with asthma, skin rashes — especially eczema, facial swelling (angioneurotic oedema), psychiatric disturbances, migraine and cot deaths in babies. Evidence for a close association between many of these disorders and food allergy is lacking, largely because tests for food allergy are not very sensitive.

Some people suffer from abdominal bloating and discomfort after taking sugars, because the sugar digesting substances (enzymes) are missing from the intestinal lining. This so-called disaccharride intolerance (the commonest is lactose intolerance; lactose is a type of sugar in milk) may be inherited but may also be caused by temporary damage to the intestine following infection or inflammation.

Can cancer affect the bowels?

Yes, but cancerous growths in the small intestine are extremely rare. This is not, however, the case in the large intestine, in which cancer is common and becoming increasingly so, in recent years. It is important to diagnose large intestinal (colonic) cancer at an early stage since it can often be cured completely by surgery. No definite causes have been found for colonic cancer, but it is believed that a low bulk diet may predispose and it has also been suggested that some food preservatives in meat may be involved as well. Many cancers form from protrusions which develop inside the bowel wall (polyps). These may sometimes cause symptoms but are often discovered incidentally in a patient being investigated for other reasons.

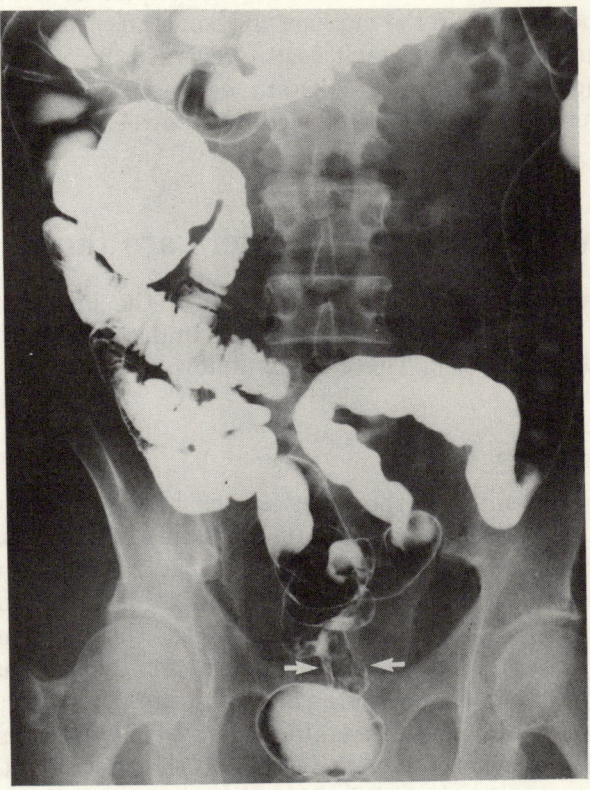

Fig. 6 A barium X-ray of the large intestine. This is narrowed in the lower part (as indicated by the arrows) due to bowel cancer. This caused bleeding from the back passage and constipation.

Symptoms of bowel cancer usually depend on which part of the large intestine is involved. On the right side, in the caecum, they are often 'silent' and may first draw attention by causing slow bleeding which results in anaemia. This is why anyone with certain types of anaemia is carefully investigated to exclude a 'silent' early cancer as being the cause. More commonly, the cancer grows into the hollow lumen or inside of the bowel from the wall and interferes with normal intestinal function. It then usually causes a change in normal bowel habit, either increasing constipation, or bouts of diarrhoea, blood in the motions and sometimes slime (mucus), abdominal pain and weight loss. Cancers in the rectum (back passage) often cause a constant desire to open the bowel (tenesmus) which is not relieved by a bowel action (defaecation).

What other bowel disorders are there?

A great number of other disorders of the intestines can occur which are less common and important than those already mentioned. These are as follows:

Ischaemic colitis

With hardening of the arteries, the blood supply to the intestine may become inadequate. If this is a slow process intestinal 'angina', pain coming on after meals, can result. Alternatively, the blood supply to the intestine may be suddenly cut off. In these circumstances, the intestine can simply become inflamed resulting in abdominal pain and the passage of blood through the back passage. This may slowly improve by itself because alternative blood channels open up over a matter of days and weeks. If the affected intestine becomes totally deprived of blood (gangrenous) this causes intense shock and peritonitis. This latter situation is very serious and the only treatment is urgent surgery.

Intussusception

This is where one portion of bowel slides inside another portion. This causes intestinal blockage and may lead to gangrene of part of the bowel. It most commonly occurs in children although there is usually no obvious reason. It does also, however, occur in adults because of a co-existent polyp or cancer. It causes abdominal pain and sometimes the passage of blood through the back passage, together with vomiting. It may settle spontaneously without surgery but operation is often necessary to correct it. In babies, it is recognised by a sudden agonised cry and the appearance of a lump in the tummy (abdomen). Sometimes after this, a 'red-currant' stool may be passed.

Volvulus

This condition occurs when a loop of bowel twists upon itself. This may happen for a number of reasons, but it is often because of scarring resulting from previous operations. It causes abdominal pain, disturbance of normal bowel function and sometimes vomiting.

Meckel's diverticulum

This is a structure like the appendix which develops from the small intestine in some people. It may become inflamed and cause very similar symptoms to appendicitis. Alternatively slow, recurrent bleeding can occur from it.

Hernias

Weaknesses can develop in the tummy (abdominal) wall most commonly in the groin regions, because of physical strains (rupture), obesity, continuous coughing or a pre-existing weakness. Through this weakness, the bowel can then intermittently protrude. This is often inconvenient and unpleasant and the sufferer may have to physically push back the bowel into the abdomen to relieve the discomfort. This is most often easily done lying down, relaxed and flat on the back. Occasionally, the bowel can become trapped. This is most common in the small groin hernias often seen in women who are overweight (femoral hernias) and gangrene or obstruction of the bowel can then occur, which requires urgent surgical treatment. Although a hernia is usually due to a portion of the bowel pushing out through a weakness in the tummy muscles, they seldom, if ever, cause disturbance of the bowel unless other complications occur.

2. WHAT IS CONSTIPATION?

How often should my bowels work?

Most people are largely unaware of the frequency of their bowel motions and overconcern with the regularity of bowel actions is not generally a good thing. Everybody has his or her own individual bowel habit and this differs from person to person. The majority of people open their bowels once a day, but to do so more or less frequently than this does not necessarily mean that anything is wrong. It may be entirely normal to evacuate the bowels as little as once a week but most people have their bowels open if not every day at least every 2nd or 3rd day. At least a quarter of people have more than one bowel action each day whereas only about one out of a hundred have an action less frequently than three times a week — but this is normal, even if uncommon. Most people's bowel habit remains fairly constant throughout their lives and the pattern they adopt happens to suit them. A pattern which remains unaltered whatever it is like within reason, seldom indicates disease, but a *change* from the normal bowel habit may well do so, unless a change in life style has also occurred.

All of these facts and figures only take into account the number of times one goes but what is also important is whether you have to strain and what is produced. Opening the bowels is an entirely normal event and the procedure itself once started is almost automatic. It should not be necessary to regularly have to strain in order to open the bowels. Similarly, passing a very small stool after a distressing degree of straining can hardly be regarded as normal, even if a bowel action by these means occurs once a day. On the other hand a person who has persistent urgency of defaecation (opening the bowels) and has to always rush to the toilet, cannot be regarded as normal either, although the number of times that the person goes each day may not be excessive. The most 'normal' estimation one can have is to pass a well formed, soft motion, effortlessly once a day, usually in the morning after breakfast. If this isn't you however, you do not necessarily have to worry, because only a proportion, even if it is a large number, of normal people do in fact do that. Any change from the normal routine, or the additional passage of blood or slime should alert you to the possibility of disease of the bowels, which can only be ruled out by seeing your doctor.

What makes my bowels sluggish?

Firstly, it is worth thinking about what makes the bowels work normally. The large bowel or colon, has been likened to a railway siding in which three trucks stand. Every day a new one arrives and bumps off the end one, so that three remain. Occasionally, one arrives with such force that it bumps off all three of them and then three days have to elapse before the siding is full enough again, so that the next truck arriving at one end can push one out at the other. Unfortunately, in real life this rather oversimplifies the situation, but it does help to illustrate just how wrong it can be to take laxatives. Following excessive or unnecessary laxatives, the bowels may be entirely emptied and will not therefore need to work normally again or cannot work for several days, until they are filled up again. Laxatives taken unnecessarily by normal people can therefore totally disturb the normal functioning of the bowel and the use of laxatives in normal people is illogical, meddlesome and potentially harmful. Emptying of the bowel is controlled by movements of the colon. This movement is triggered normally by a number of different things, namely: *(1) Eating* — when food or drink enters the stomach, this fires a direct reflex or signal to the bowel to start activity. This is the warning in the railway siding that another truck is on its way! It explains why it is common to need to open the bowels after a meal, especially the first one of the day. *(2) Movement* — changing position, standing up, walking, running and any physical activity, all stimulate the bowel into action. Constipation commonly occurs in invalids confined to bed and normal people who get constipated are often not very active. *(3) Emotion* — Both stress and emotional situations can have profound effects on the movements of the bowel, most commonly to increase the frequency of bowel actions. We all know what stress, such as a job interview or speaking in public can do to the bowels! On the other hand, mental depression not uncommonly causes constipation. Usually, sleep (a time deprived of emotion and motion!) slows the bowel down.

Consequently, changes in any of the normal daily activities can have dramatic effects on the bowels.

Why me?

The commonest cause of constipation is in part, due to the rush of modern life. The call or desire to go to the lavatory is ignored, so that a bus or train can be caught. Other reasons for neglecting the urge to open the bowels are laziness, a chilly, smelly or filthy lavatory, false modesty if the lavatory is in a place where everybody 'knows' that you have gone to it or you can be 'overheard' in, or painful piles. Holidays and times spent away from home make people forget, because they have other interests and become distracted or there is a queue for the toilet. It is most commonly this and not the change of water that causes constipation on holiday!

Repeatedly ignoring the call to stool, means that the normal mechanisms responsible for opening the bowels 'switch off' and do not respond to the messages to do so as they would normally. Often bad habits in childhood are carried over into adult life and constant ignoring of the desire to defaecate becomes a way of life, so that the bowels become permanently lazy and sluggish. Other factors which interfere with the normal nerve mechanisms responsible for opening the bowels are, lack of physical activity or food. Food usually stimulates activity of the bowels but is less likely to do so when a person is lying down. Invalids often suffer this way and additionally the need to bother someone else to get a bedpan or commode often further aggravates the situation. It is also natural for the bowels not to open regularly when a person stops eating, especially during an illness, when days may pass without the desire to open the bowels. Astronauts in space only need to open their bowels about once or twice a week. This is not because they are not eating, it is just that they eat food which contains virtually no residue or waste and there is little material left over to form faeces.

For these reasons, it is not at all uncommon for anyone to become constipated who does not eat regularly and well (roughage-containing foods) or who does not exercise frequently. These are the usual reasons why anyone ill in bed becomes constipated and it is often made worse in people who are depressed or have other nervous illnesses, although the reasons for this are by no means clear.

Modern toilet seats may also be a factor in developing bad bowel habits. The most natural way to open the bowels is probably in the squatting position, as natives do in the jungle! This position is almost impossible on a modern high toilet seat, especially if the feet do not rest firmly on the ground. Children should not be allowed to sit on the toilet with legs dangling but should be encouraged to use a foot stool. Once again, anyone who is ill is at a disadvantage if they are unable to get to a toilet. Using a bedpan means one has to adopt about the most unnatural position of all, and whenever possible an elderly of infirm person should be allowed the use of a commode and if possible in private!

Women tend to be the most frequent sufferers from constipation and it is normal in some for the bowel function to vary during the monthly (menstrual) cycle. Over one half of women notice a change in bowel habit at the time of the monthly period and although most suffer from the passage of loose stools, about one in eight experience constipation. It is not known why this is, but it has been suggested that hormone changes are important.

Some drugs also cause constipation as a side effect of their use. Although many do this, the most frequent offenders are pain-killers containing codeine and antacids made with aluminium compounds.

Is it a disease?

Constipation in itself is not a disease and in most people who consider themselves 'constipated' it does not signify anything abnormal. It can, however, in some cases accompany an underlying disorder.

Constipation with variable amounts of abdominal pain occurs in people suffering from an *irritable colon* or *diverticular disease*. Constipation in these conditions may imply infrequent bowel actions but more commonly, difficulty in passing hard, pellet-like stools. Diverticular disease is commoner the older the person, but an irritable colon can occur at almost any age. Mucus discharge with bowel motions, the passage of lots of wind or flatus through the back passage and abdominal bloating or distension may also occur in these conditions.

Constipation also occurs in *megacolon (Hirschsprung's disease)*. In this rare condition, some of the nervous connections to the bowel do not fully develop and the bowel does not function normally. Because of this, evacuation is incomplete and with time, the bowel gets progressively larger and the patient more and more constipated. Most sufferer's develop problems in childhood, although this can be a cause of constipation in later life. Because of the loss of normal bowel control an individual with this condition may not only become constipated but also lose voluntary control of bowel evacuation and become incontinent, leading to faecal soiling. The same sometimes occurs in elderly people who suffer from constipation. Liquid motions bypass hard (impacted) faeces and spill out uncontrollably as diarrhoea.

Women often become constipated in *pregnancy* and although it is not fully understood why this should be, hormonal changes that occur in pregnancy are assumed to play a part.

One of the first symptoms of *bowel cancer* can be constipation. The normal bowel habit commonly changes and increasing constipation develops which may necessitate the use of laxatives to overcome it. It may be this which leads to another common symptom which is alternating episodes of constipation and diarrhoea, sometimes accompanied by rectal bleeding and griping pain in the abdomen.

Sufferers from *piles* and *anal fissures* often become constipated because evacuation of the bowels causes pain. This often leads to deliberately avoiding responding to the call to stool and this commonly results in a vicious circle of constipation, because the stool becomes increasingly hard and so more difficult and painful to pass.

Constipation can also occur due to a number of *other disorders* including an underactive thyroid, depression and mental illnesses, damage to the bowel by previous overusage of laxatives and also by drugs used to treat other diseases.

Does constipation cause pain?

When somebody is constipated, the bowel can become distended and this may be uncomfortable. Passing infrequent, hard stools also aggravates haemorrhoids and anal fissures, which can cause pain in or around the back passage.

Pain in the abdomen together with constipation are most commonly due to bowel spasm in sufferers from an irritable bowel or diverticular disease, or due to obstruction of the bowel which can occur in intestinal inflammation or cancer.

Bowel spasm can cause pain anywhere in the abdomen. It is often a griping or colicky pain which comes and goes in waves but it can also be an intense, nagging discomfort. Most commonly the pain is felt in the left lower part of the abdomen above the groin or alternatively centrally below the umbilicus or navel. It is often made better by opening the bowels or the use of drugs which relieve spasm (anti-spasmodics) but usually not much else helps.

Pain due to obstruction of the bowel by an intestinal cancer or any other cause such as inflammation may be very similar. It is only possible in most cases to exclude cancer by the appropriate tests and anybody who experiences constant, severe pain in the tummy or recurrent pains with bowel upset should see a doctor.

Does regular use of my bowels make me any healthier?

There is no known connection between regular bowels motions and good health or the opposite, irregular bowels and poor health. However, constipation can occur as a result of some other illnesses and is often caused by a less than perfect life-style. Although for centuries there has been a general belief that regular use of the bowels leads to better health and this philosophy underlies many herbal remedies, there is absolutely no proof of this. It has been suggested in the past that poisons of some sort are absorbed into the bloodstream if the bowels are not opened daily and there is a certain element of truth in this. However, no toxins or poisons from the motions are known to be absorbed that can cause headaches, bad breath or lethargy as some people believe. Bacteria do live in the normal bowel and some of them produce ammonia and bad smelling gases that do enter the bloodstream. The gases may then escape from the body on the breath and a build up of ammonia can be serious in sufferers from liver disease but there is nothing to suggest that regular emptying of the bowels is of any benefit to the health of normal people.

Is there anything I can do to regulate my bowels?

A belief in the 'purifying' properties of a purge has existed since ancient times. This is nonsense, but many people still believe it when they take a laxative (a chemical which stimulates movement of the bowel) or dose of 'liver-salts', or give these to their children. Advertisements designed to sell purgatives (something that makes the stool loose) have generally misled many people into taking laxatives in the belief that regular use of the bowels is essential in order to keep fit and healthy. It is not at all uncommon for people to have grown up with the idea that missing a bowel action is serious and that symptoms of being run down are due to this, since purgatives have been suggested as a cure for many illnesses from the earliest times. So a purge is taken, which often empties the entire gut and several days pass before a normal motion can form again. Putting this down to constipation, the victims purge themselves again and again and sooner or later a purge is relied upon regularly to open the bowels. This may be good business for manufacturers of laxatives but long-term use can be very dangerous since the bowels may become seriously damaged.

The most effective ways of treating constipation are often the simplest. Prevention is the best remedy and avoiding the factors that cause constipation most important; especially poor toilet facilities, late rising and the rush to get to school or work, shift working, lack of physical exercise, rushed and irregular meals and food with little or no roughage.

The natural constituent of the diet which is lacking so often is fibre or roughage that adds bulk. The bulkier the motion, the more the bowel is stimulated to work regularly. Considerable roughage should be eaten in everybody's diet and there are few exceptions. The most suitable foods are fresh vegetables and fruit which are only lightly cooked or eaten raw, wholemeal and wholewheat bread and bran (a by-product of the milling of wheat which contains cellulose, and this is the part that has been taken out of most brown and white breads) and also many breakfast cereals (the best always carry the amount of fibre printed on the box). Never use regular laxatives even though they can be bought at the chemists without a prescription. If these simple remedies do not work and you are definitely constipated you need to consult your doctor anyway and he or she will advise you what is safe to take. Special problems often exist in children, old people and during pregnancy as far as constipation is concerned. The simple principles of prevention and treatment are, however, similar in all of these instances and failure of these simple remedies necessitates consultation with your doctor. The most important thing that you can do in any case is to stay regular and not to miss or put off the call to pass a stool.

3. WHAT OTHER BOWEL DISTURBANCES ARE THERE?

How do I know if I've got bowel trouble?

Apart from the intestines, other parts of the digestive system are in the tummy region as are many other internal organs including the kidneys, bladder, spleen and in women the womb. Problems occurring in any of these organs can give rise to very similar symptoms and people often find it difficult to pinpoint their own aches and pains. It is worth bearing in mind the following common digestive symptoms:

Coating of the tongue is usually due to poor oral hygiene (cleansing of the mouth), lack of chewing of food or breathing through the mouth. It is usually due to one or other of these causes but is also seen in debilitating illnesses.

Halitosis or bad breath often occurs in similar circumstances. It is usually aggravated by eating spiced foods especially curries and garlic and some gases formed within the intestine may also be passed out (excreted) on the breath and produce a bad smell. This is especially so when fat in the diet is digested. Some of the partly digested fat (call fatty acids) enters the blood stream and evaporates on the breath to give halitosis. This will often be improved if the amount of fat in the diet is reduced. People with stomach ailments which cause hold-up of the stomach contents also have halitosis as do people with bad teeth.

Heartburn (a burning discomfort felt behind the breast-bone — also called the sternum) is usually due to inflammation of the gullet lining (oesophagitis) and sometimes also associated with bitter acid entering the mouth.

Vomiting is usually due to many minor things but can be caused by inflammation or ulceration of the stomach, oesophagus or duodenum. It also occurs with cancerous growths in the stomach or oesophagus. It may also be due to many other causes including, rarely, kidney failure, brain tumours or hormonal disturbances. Medical treatment, particularly aspirin and anti-inflammatory drugs, also commonly causes nausea, vomiting, heartburn and indigestion.

Hiccups are due to repetitive contractions of the diaphragm (the muscles separating the chest from the tummy). This may be due to irritation of the nerve supply to these muscles, drugs, kidney failure or a number of other causes, but usually there is no obvious cause. There is no particularly effective treatment apart from the usual well-known remedies.

Dyspepsia (indigestion) usually implies upper abdominal burning discomfort and may be related to food. This is most often not due to any serious disease but alcohol, a stomach ulcer, inflammation of the stomach, duodenum or oesophagus or gallstones may cause it.

Gut bleeding may result in vomiting fresh blood, altered blood (usually looking like coffee-grounds) or passing partly digested blood in the stools (melaena) which looks like jet-black tar and has a distinctive, unpleasant smell. The usual causes are stomach ulcers or growths, inflammation of the stomach by drugs, especially aspirin, or bleeding from the gullet. The latter is most commonly due to a tear of the gullet lining, sometimes brought on by vomiting or retching, or varicose veins in the gullet (oesophagus) due to liver disease. Bleeding is a serious problem requiring hospital observation and treatment.

Iron tablets for anaemia and some stomach medicines also turn the stools black but this is not due to bleeding.

Weight loss in the absence of an obvious cause, such as a reduced diet or increased exercise, usually requires investigation. It may be due to a 'silent' stomach ulcer or growth in the digestive system, bowel disease or an hormonal imbalance, usually an overactive thyroid.

Can bowel trouble cause pain?

Since the normal function of the intestine is absorption of food, intestinal disorders may interfere with this and prevent food absorption which can lead to diarrhoea. Blowing up (distension) or irritation (spasm) of the bowel causes pain. Many disorders, particularly those due to spasm, inflammation or cancers, cause obstruction to the hollow lumen or inside of the intestine which causes distension. This can be painful and may be worsened if the normal movements of the bowel (peristalsis) attempt to overcome the problem. This can cause pain to come in waves (colic) and be griping in nature.

Pain from the small intestine is often in the centre of the abdomen, that from the large bowel usually but not always, around the outer part of the abdomen. Complete obstruction of the intestine may cause vomiting, pain, loss of fluid from the body (dehydration) and failure of normal intestinal function — with either diarrhoea or constipation — with the complete absence of the passage of faeces or wind.

Severe abdominal pain

Any severe, persistent pain requires urgent medical attention. There are innumerable causes and these can only be discovered by prompt examination and appropriate investigations.

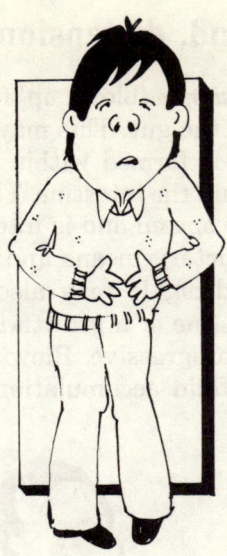

What is colic due to then?

'Colic' means blockage of one of the many hollow tubes within the abdomen. It is typically waves of pain which are griping in nature, building up over a few minutes to a crescendo, easing for a time and then starting again. True colic which is persistent, is usually due to blockage of an internal organ and is likely to require hospital treatment. This may be because of gallstones, when in the right upper part of the abdomen and going through to the back, kidney stones if in the flank and going down to the groin, or obstruction of the intestine if centrally placed in the abdomen. Gallstones may also cause jaundice, kidney stones, blood in the urine together with urinary frequency and intestinal obstruction, vomiting and bowel disturbance — usually diarrhoea but sometimes constipation. Spasm of the bowel may also cause a similar type of discomfort.

33

What about wind, distension and gurgling?

Abdominal distension (a 'blown up' feeling) is usually due to excess gas within the gut. This may be swallowed, in an anxious individual, or formed within the gut by bacteria fermenting food within the intestine. This frequently occurs in people with bowel spasm and is intermittent and can be settled usually by dietary means and drugs which relieve spasm (anti-spasmodics). It may also indicate an actual blockage of the intestine or a growth in the tummy region and is then usually progressive. Blowing up of the tummy can also be due to fluid accumulation caused by liver or heart disease.

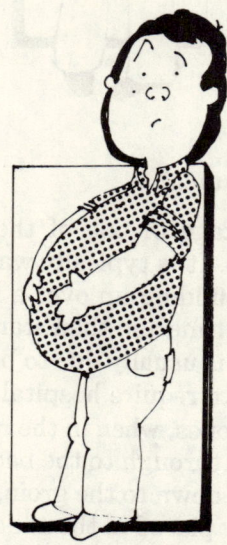

Flatulence (passage of wind) is a normal occurrence. It is usually brought up in an attempt to reduce abdominal discomfort or distension. Most gas burped is originally swallowed. Several types of gas form in the intestines. Nitrogen, oxygen, carbon dioxide, hydrogen and methane are the important ones but ammonia and hydrogen sulphide are also present. Most that is produced within the bowel is as a result of fermentation of food by bacteria but some is swallowed. The normal bowel contains about 150 ml of gas and yet about ten times this is produced daily. Some is reabsorbed into the body but the remainder is passed out as flatus ('wind'). Most normal people probably pass flatus a dozen times a day. It is well known that certain foods make considerably more wind than others. Carbohydrates (sugars and starch), legumes principally beans (which can increase wind production 6-fold), wheat and also broccoli, brussels sprouts, cabbage and particularly root vegetables such as turnips, swedes and artichokes are the worst offenders. Too much fibre in the diet can also do the same. Considerable wind may also in rare cases imply a digestive abnormality causing sugars to be improperly digested and allowing them passage into the large intestine. Lack of milk digesting chemicals or enzymes is a common cause of this and reduction in the amount of milk in the diet or these other foods can be helpful. Excessive overactivity of the bowel, as occurs in an irritable colon due to irritability or actual disease of the bowel, can cause excess wind to form. Suppression of the desire to evacuate the gas can cause abdominal bloating and discomfort. Obviously custom dictates whether or not flatus is passed in public and by and large men tend to be more liberal in their outlook than women in this regard! It is probably because women are reluctant to pass wind that they tend to suffer more from bloating and abdominal discomfort than men. It is something that society has changed its attitudes to over the centuries. In Elizabethan days passing wind in public was commonplace. However this pastimes caused public offence in Ancient Rome until the Emperor Claudius issue an edict to permit the escape of wind and made this lawful for all Romans!

Infantile colic, a frequent cause of constant screaming in babies is often due to flatulence as can be seen since it is often relieved when flatus is passed.

If excessive, the symptoms can usually be reduced by

altering the diet, a mild sedative or an anti-spasmodic. Eating charcoal biscuits may also reduce some abdominal bloating. A moderate increase in fibre in the diet can be helpful in reducing the amount of wind and also improving the odour of flatus and stools. Eating orange peel may also be of value in improving the smell!

Audible gurgling (borborygmi) is usually associated with these other symptoms and due to similar causes. It is produced by contractions of loops of intestine containing both fluid and gas. It is, of course, normal to hear a few 'rumblings' throughout the day but especially when hungry and just before a meal. If excessive, it may be because of some obstruction to the intestines.

This combination of complaints (rumblings and wind) has been called burbulence by the American poet Ogden Nash!

What is meant by diarrhoea?

Diarrhoea means the need to pass frequent, loose motions. Opening of the bowels more than once a day may or may not be due to disease. Obviously if it is associated with other symptoms such as blood or slime in the motions, abdominal pain, weight loss, persistent mouth ulcers, anaemia or general ill-health you should see your doctor. Often it will be due to bowel irritability but this can only be determined by investigation. Other features such as bulky, offensively smelling stools which have been difficult to flush away in the toilet and float in the lavatory pan may indicate a digestive abnormality. However, especially in adolescents there are usually other obvious causes in the absence of additional symptoms, for increased frequency of bowel action. Women in their reproductive period of life not infrequently have increased frequency of bowel action at the time of their periods. Young male adolescents may imbibe large quantities of beer which can cause diarrhoea — especially 'real' ale! A change in bowel habit, being woken at night by the need to open the bowels or other constitutional disturbances (signs of ill-health) are usually symptoms suggestive of disease. The failure to get better when the amount of fibre in the diet is increased may also be reason for further investigations. Some drugs, particularly magnesium-containing antacids and antibiotics, can also cause loose motions.

Faecal soiling (incontinence of faeces)

This complaint is a great deal commoner than is usually thought and can sometimes be confused with diarrhoea. It is often due to liquid motion leaking uncontrollably from the back passage and soiling the clothes and is of course very distressing. It can be due to many different problems. It may occur in someone who is very constipated and the response of the bowel to overcome this or the frequent use of purgatives means that very loose motions can spill from the anus. Usually the back passage remains tightly closed by the combined effects of muscular contractions. If these muscles are damaged (perhaps in childbirth or an accident) or the nerves are affected in any way, these normal controls may be ineffective.

This particular problem may be difficult to treat but this can often be done after careful investigation of the cause. Since someone suffering from this trouble is often naturally embarrassed by it or confuses it with diarrhoea it really is important to explain to your doctor what exactly is troubling you.

What could cause my diarrhoea?

With most people who suffer a short period of frequent loose bowel motions it is usually due either to dietary indiscretion or gastroenteritis (food poisoning). Everybody can be upset occasionally by 'rich' foods and curries are notorious for upsetting those unused to them. Any normal person can, if they eat enough food especially that containing fat, overload the digestive processes and get diarrhoea. Arctic explorers often eat considerable amounts of fatty foods to maintain their body warmth, and 'body-builders' eat meat to build up muscles and both of these groups of people suffer on occasions from loose motions because of this. Gastroenteritis due to inflammation of the digestive system caused by infection also often causes bowel upset. The infection usually enters the body from drinking dirty water or eating food that has 'gone off' and infection of the stomach often causes vomiting to start with, sometimes within hours or if not a day or two. Soon after this because the infection moves down to the intestines, griping tummy ache (abdominal colic) begins and diarrhoea soon follows. The afflicted person usually feels terrible for a few days but within a week or 10 days is fully recovered.

More long-standing diarrhoea may be due to irritability of the bowel — an irritable colon or diverticular disease. A person suffering with these disorders often needs to open the bowels several times first thing in the morning but is then reasonably well for the remainder of the day. Occasionally the need to go urgently after meals also occurs and sometimes the results are fairly 'explosive'. Undigested food ('corn on the cob' is common) can occasionally appear in the faeces. These problems may get worse when a person is under some kind of stress. It should not be forgotten that taking certain medicines also commonly causes diarrhoea.

Finally the rarer causes of diarrhoea include bowel inflammation. Coeliac disease caused by inflammation of the small intestine because of a reaction to wheat in food is an important cause. This disorder interferes with food absorption into the body. If this is severely limited, nourishment from the food may not enter the body in sufficient quantities. In children, this can interfere with growth and commonly in coeliac disease, the arms and legs become thin and spindly and yet the tummy is blown up and protuberant. In adults the same problems may occur, although loss of weight is more common and diarrhoea usually but not always occurs.

If digestion of fat is badly affected, the motions become extremely bulky and appear full of fat droplets, may be pale in colour, smell very badly and float on the water in the toilet and are extremely difficult to flush away. Other digestive disorders, including inadequate function by the pancreatic gland, may cause the same problems. The pancreas (in animals the sweet-bread) is a gland that produces two kinds of chemicals (secretion). One is insulin that controls the amount of sugar in the blood, the other the digestive juices that help to break down food in the intestines. This gland can be damaged in a number of ways, and when this happens the digestion of food is interfered with and diarrhoea results. In adults, long-standing alcohol excess causing damage and in children an inherited defect, cystic fibrosis, are amongst the commonest causes of an inadequately functioning gland. In cystic fibrosis, mucus (or slime) production throughout the body but especially in the lungs and the pancreas is abnormal. Mucus is important to protect the surface of these vital organs and in cystic fibrosis, lung and pancreas damage results. It is usually necessary to replace the absent pancreatic secretions by tablets and medicines that are swallowed, to prevent the diarrhoea and loss of nourishment from the body. The other inflammatory disorders of the gut which can cause diarrhoea are Crohn's disease and ulcerative colitis. If the inflammation in Crohn's disease affects the small intestine, griping pains and diarrhoea result, as well as loss of weight. In colitis, blood and slime mixed with the diarrhoea are most common and the same may occur in bowel cancer.

Some people who have had previous operations on the stomach in which the vagus nerve has been cut to reduce stomach acid, suffer from diarrhoea afterwards. This often comes on urgently after meals and can cause very watery diarrhoea. It can usually be controlled by antidiarrhoeal medicines or other means.

Should I see my doctor about my diarrhoea?

As with constipation the word diarrhoea means different things to different people but it is a little easier to define and most people use it to mean frequent loose motions. It is difficult to be absolutely specific about when someone with loose motions should see his or her doctor. On the whole, frequent diarrhoea normally means that there is something wrong with the bowels but it does not necessarily have be a serious disorder. The only way to be certain is by seeing your doctor. Only one out of every hundred people regularly have bowel actions more than three times each day and this is probably the best guide — anybody going this frequently should see their doctor.

Can 'nerves' cause diarrhoea?

Everybody when he or she is under any kind of tension or stress is liable to diarrhoea. Facing up to a job interview, an examination, making a speech, are all occasions which can produce a few loose motions in anybody and this is normal. People who suffer from bowel irritability are more likely to react to stress than other people and often find that being 'on edge' can easily upset the bowels. People who suffer from bowel diseases can also be upset by stress and find that their bowels get worse. Stress has even been thought in the past to cause ulcerative colitis and some other bowel diseases but this is unproven.

Is there anything I can do about diarrhoea?

Yes there is. Firstly you can try to prevent yourself catching gastroenteritis. Always wash your hands carefully before touching any food whether you are eating it or preparing it for others. It is also very important not to leave food, especially any that is not going to be cooked fully, exposed to flies that can transmit disease. The worst time of the year for this is, of course, the summer time and warm food that is left cooling or exposed to the sun is most likely to cause trouble. When you are buying food, particularly the kinds that you will eat without fully cooking (cream cakes are the worst offenders), be particular which shops you buy from. Avoid those that look dirty and have flies buzzing around. If you are travelling abroad, a lot of people believe in medicines that can be bought from the chemists to prevent diarrhoea. It has never been really convincingly shown that these work and some can be harmful — as a general rule it is better not to take any medicines unless they are absolutely necessary. If you are travelling to an exotic part of the world where they have cholera or typhoid (dysenteries) it might be worth seeing your doctor about immunisation first. Unfortunately the 'jabs' do not work in everyone and the effect is only short lived but it is certainly better than catching these infections! Some people who regularly travel to 'far-flung' parts of the world say that it is safest to buy drinks made in the local 'Coke' factory. At least these places are usually regularly inspected and are likely to be safer than some of the other local producers. Similarly it is important that food should be clean, well cooked and not saved to be eaten later. Fruit should be unblemished and washed and you should peel it yourself. Ice cream in foreign countries is usually especially suspect. Water should not be drunk unless previously boiled and/or sterilized with appropriate agents.

If you catch diarrhoea, there is not really a great deal that you can do. If you are in a hot climate, since a lot of water and salt can be lost from the body in diarrhoea, it is important to continue to drink liquids. Sugary drinks with a pinch of salt added are the best as long as they do not make you sick. Sticking to a light diet, or avoiding food for a day or two may also be helpful. Avoiding milk and milk products until the diarrhoea has settled also helps and resting in bed can make you feel better especially if you feel 'washed out'. It is better to avoid taking any sort of medicine bought from the chemist. If you are bad enough to need medicines, you really need a doctor first. As a general rule, if your diarrhoea continues for more than a week or two you should see a doctor. If you are really unwell, develop a temperature (fever) or you notice anything else, really bad stomach pains that double you up or stop you sleeping, blood mixed with the motions or sickness that stops you keeping any drink or food down for more than a day, you should also see the doctor. It is very difficult to make rules about this kind of situation but if you think that you have more than simple gastroenteritis it is best to check with a doctor, because you will not know what is going on unless you do. It is usually better to play safe than be sorry at a later date!

Finally, if you have got diarrhoea that you think is perhaps due to gastroenteritis, try and spare someone else catching it! If you are fairly certain you caught it from any particular food, warn your friends, the people selling it and if necessary the local public health inspectors — it is one of their jobs to control this sort of thing. Be especially careful if you have to prepare someone else's food and try to avoid doing this, if you can, until you are better. Wash your hands very thoroughly, especially after going to the toilet, and use disposable crockery and cutlery until you are better or keep a set for your own use that other people will not use. If you handle food for others, or if a child at school is affected it is best to stay away from work or school until the diarrhoea has gone away. Try especially to avoid any direct contact with susceptible individuals — the very young and the elderly. These are the people who are most likely to suffer serious consequences from gastroenteritis.

Diarrhoea should be taken most seriously in the very young (less than five years old, especially in the first 6 months of life) and the elderly (over 65 years old). Children or elderly people who are constipated not uncommonly develop diarrhoea when the faeces become so-called 'impacted'. This means that the constipation becomes sufficiently severe for the bowel to attempt to overcome it by producing copious watery secretions which bypass the hard constipated stools and cause diarrhoea. Diarrhoea should also be taken seriously in anybody with any other significant medical problem, especially diabetes.

4. WHAT CAN I DO FOR MY BOWELS?

What should I do about my life-style?

Many disorders of the digestive system are caused by various aspects of modern living and some can therefore be prevented. Improved standards of hygiene, clean water and good food have reduced infections of the intestine in the Western world, but our current life styles have brought their own problems.

Diet

Taking small, frequent, nutritious meals is probably the greatest favour you can do your bowels. Big eaters almost invariably have loose bowels presumably because the sheer size of meals poses an excessive stimulus to the normal mechanisms controlling the intestines. Eating large quantities of highly processed and refined foods (so-called 'junk foods') especially white bread, cakes, pastries, biscuits, crisps and chips are widely believed to be the cause of a number of digestive disorders, in particular bowel irritability, diverticular disease and possibly bowel cancer. The fibre content of the diet should be fairly high and this is best achieved with bran, All Bran, muesli, wholewheat or wholemeal bread, fruit and lightly cooked or uncooked fresh vegetables.

Some chemical components of food, especially nitrites in preserved meats and bacon, are suspected by some to play a role in the development of bowel cancer, although this is not proven.

Few digestive conditions benefit from specific dietary exclusion. In coeliac disease withdrawal of gluten from the diet is essential. Other people have inadequate intestinal chemicals to digest milk and sometimes sugars. Some patients with ulcerative colitis or even with gastroenteritis will benefit from milk withdrawal. It has been suggested that Prince Charles Edward the Stuart Pretender to the Throne (Bonnie Prince Charlie) may have suffered from ulcerative colitis (all such problems at that time were collectively known as the 'bloody flux'!). Shortly after the Battle of Culloden in 1746 he was afflicted and is reported to have cured himself in three days by excluding milk from his diet! Other patients definitely suffer from allergy to foods but most of these are difficult to identify properly. Apart from avoiding foods which are known to cause symptoms, very few people otherwise benefit from cutting out any particular items.

It should also be remembered that some foods contain natural compounds which can affect gut movement, such as onions, and lead to heartburn or loose motions and wind. Others, especially baked beans and also bran, can lead to excess gas formation which causes gaseous distension and discomfort in some individuals. Other foods especially rhubarb and prunes, contain chemicals which are natural aperients that stimulate the bowels and can cause diarrhoea. Tannin in tea tends to constipate although if milk is added this perhaps partly neutralizes the effect, whereas coffee has a laxative effect probably because it contains caffeine.

Temperature

Temperature also influences bowel activity. Hot drinks stimulate the bowels but warmth applied to the abdominal skin (such as with a hot water bottle) tends to soothe abdominal colic. On the other hand, a cold bath each morning was strongly recommended at the turn of the last century as a stimulus for daily bowel action and a cold drink probably has a similar effect.

Exercise

Regular exercise is helpful since it stimulates bowel movements and reduces any tendency to constipation. In the past, massage has also been advocated to have this effect. One such recommendation a hundred years ago, was to roll a cannon-ball weighing up to 10 pounds and covered in chamois-leather over the abdomen along the probable course of the colon!

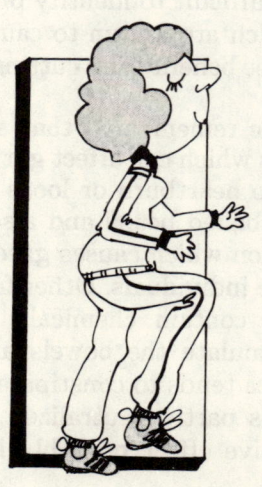

Smoking

Smoking normally provokes the call to stool. This may help constipated individuals but can make matters worse for someone with diarrhoea. This is probably due to the nicotine in tobacco smoke. If this is relied upon to regularly open the bowels, giving up smoking is not uncommonly followed by a period of constipation. It has been recently shown that only a very small number of patients with ulcerative colitis regularly smoke. No one knows why this is but, it has even been suggested that smoking and the use of nicotine-chewing gum may be beneficial to some people with colitis!

Why does everybody talk so much about diet nowadays?

Well, what we all eat in this day and age is really a very experimental diet in terms of the development of the human race. We haven't been eating it for very long at all, although many of us may have been brought up on the kinds of food we now eat regularly. It is worth remembering that the food we consume is very different from that enjoyed by our grandparents. Because of the demands placed on the food industry over the past few decades, the preparation and presentation of our food has changed dramatically. Intensive farming methods mean that we eat meat which has a very different composition to that produced at the turn of the last century. The need for the transportation and preservation of a huge amount and variety of different foods has necessitated the use of preserving methods, the long term consequences of which nobody has any idea about. What is more, the pattern of our eating has also altered enormously. It has been estimated for example that 200 years ago the average person consumed six pounds of sugar each year. 100 years ago this had increased four times and today most people get through 120–150 pounds of sugar each year.

Along with this dramatic increase in sugar consumption, grain cereals have been deprived of the fibrous coating before arriving at our breakfast table and the use of white-flour products has become extremely widespread. We know as an example that this alteration in eating pattern has had a measurable effect on the amount of stomach acid we make and this may play a part in causing stomach ulcers. We also know that changes in diet influence the normal movements of the intestines and the bacteria which normally live within the bowels but many of the other possible effects of dietary change are unknown and remain speculative.

What is wrong with what I eat already?

If there is such a thing as the average British diet it probably consists of a number of the following: white bread, cornflakes, eggs, cheese, cakes, biscuits, chocolates, pies, chips and potatoes, frozen vegetables and tinned fruit. On top of that we drink tea, coffee, coridals, alcohol and water. We consume 2000–2500 calories of energy, 100 grams of fat, 70–80 grams of protein each day and this diet also contains 300 grams of carbohydrate, including 2–3 ounces of sugar each day. What does this all mean in practice? Firstly, since most of us are fairly sedentary and inactive, this is more than our bodies actually need. Secondly, this average diet only contains a little less than 20 grams of dietary fibre each day (one third coming from cereals and the remainder from fruit and vegetables) which is about half of what we actually need. In its place we imbibe nutrients we do not particularly require (for instance in the form of alcohol) even if we do like them! 80% of men in our society regularly drink alcohol and, on average, consume 1½ pints each day of the year!

What can I do about the food I eat?

A more sensible diet as far as the needs of our body are concerned, would include wholemeal bread, fibre-containing cereals (Weetabix, All Bran, Shredded Wheat) and biscuits (bran or digestive), chicken, fish, fresh fruit and vegetables, clear and home-made soups and jacket potatoes. The main purpose of this kind of dietary change is to reduce the amount of fat and the proportion of fat in the diet as well as salt and alcohol, and to increase carbohydrate as an energy source (but the kind of carbohydrate that is not 'refined' such as sugar). The best way that this can be achieved is to decrease fat by halving the amount of butter and margarine spread on bread, by eating lean in preference to the fatty meats such as pork and lamb, and by eating fewer sausages and preserved meats. Cream should be reserved for special occasions only, high fat (gold top) milk avoided, with perhaps skimmed milk used instead and the amount of cheese eaten halved. Eating more bread (wholemeal) increases the amount of carbohydrate as does more breakfast cereal and starchy vegetables, especially potatoes, but you should not increase the amount of milk and sugar taken with cereals.

You should eat regular meals. Frequent small meals are probably the most beneficial, rather than sitting down and gorging at irregular intervals or eating snacks between meals. Do not overeat at meal times and try to leave the table when you are still able to eat more. Eat breakfast each day.

The main problem is that this will probably cost appreciably more than you have been used to spending on your food unless you also cut down on the amount of meat eaten. I am afraid that there is little that can be done about that but, just because you may not have to think about your body and what to feed it very often, isn't it still very important to you? After all, it is the only one you've got and you look after your car and house, don't you?

What foods should I eat for my bowels?

The simple answer for most people is to eat more dietary fibre. This is especially important to anybody with constipation, especially in pregnancy or for children, anyone with an irritable colon, diverticular disease, piles (haemorrhoids) and fissures and probably also Crohn's disease. Very few doctors nowadays would recommend low residue diets.

The simplest way of doing this is by eating fibre-containing cereal foods and wholemeal bread, but you should only eat the right amounts and the quantity depends on each individual. Lightly cooked or raw fruit and vegetables also contain useful amounts of fibre but oat-based cereals, including porridge, are on the whole, less effective. Eat the skins of fruit. Dried fruit, and nuts can also help. As a rough guide, you should probably double the amount of fibre in your diet if you are not already eating a special high

Food	Fibre content (grams)
Wholemeal bread — 6 slices	20
Brown bread — 6 slices	9
2 Weetabix/Shredded Wheat	6
Similar portion of All-Bran	10
Large helping of: beans (broad beans or baked beans) or peas	5
Rye crispbread — slice	5
Large banana	4
Large apple/pear/orange	2

fibre diet, and aim at eating 40 grams of fibre each day. The table will give you some idea of the amount of fibre present in normal size portions of common foods.

What is roughage?

It is the fibre contained within the food we eat. This is the skeleton (or scaffolding) that supports plants. It is this skeleton that holds plants together and gives them shape and strength. Within the fibrous skeleton are the cells containing nourishment and the protective shell has to be broken down before your body can use the nutrients. Your body will do this anyway when you eat vegetables and fruit, although the process is already started if these are first cooked (and some of the nutrients are lost in cooking anyway). Most of the fibre is destroyed by overcooking or removed in modern food processing.

Fibre is a mixture of relatively indestructible substances, most of which when eaten pass through the digestive system largely unchanged and undigested. In the digestive system fibre softens the stools, making them more easily passed and preventing constipation, and it increases the bulk of the food residue passing through the intestines by acting like a sponge, trapping fluid and gases as it goes along. This gives the bowel more soft matter to push along and means that it does not have to push so hard. Because of this, less pressure builds up inside the bowel which might otherwise cause weaknesses to develop in the bowel wall as occurs in diverticular disease. As a result, there will not be discomfort as happens because of spasm in people with irritable bowels. Fibre also changes the numbers and types of bacteria in the bowel which can help to reduce the numbers of toxic substances present within the bowels and this probably helps to prevent bowel cancer. Finally fibre lessens the amount of energy contained inside food entering the body by reducing the amount absorbed from the intestines. It also requires more chewing and digestion. Because of this you can eat less and feel fuller and yet, since less food is absorbed, you should not gain weight.

If you decide to increase the amount of fibre in your diet you can easily do this by eating ordinary foods that contain roughage. A lot of people will have been told about bran. There is nothing magical about this, but it is simply a type of food that contains a high proportion of fibre. If it suits you, well that is fine, but many people do not like it. If you don't, there is no need to worry, lots of other foods contain roughage but you may just have to eat more of them. If you do decide to eat bran, then raw, unprocessed bran is more effective than cooked bran (as in breakfast cereals) and coarse,

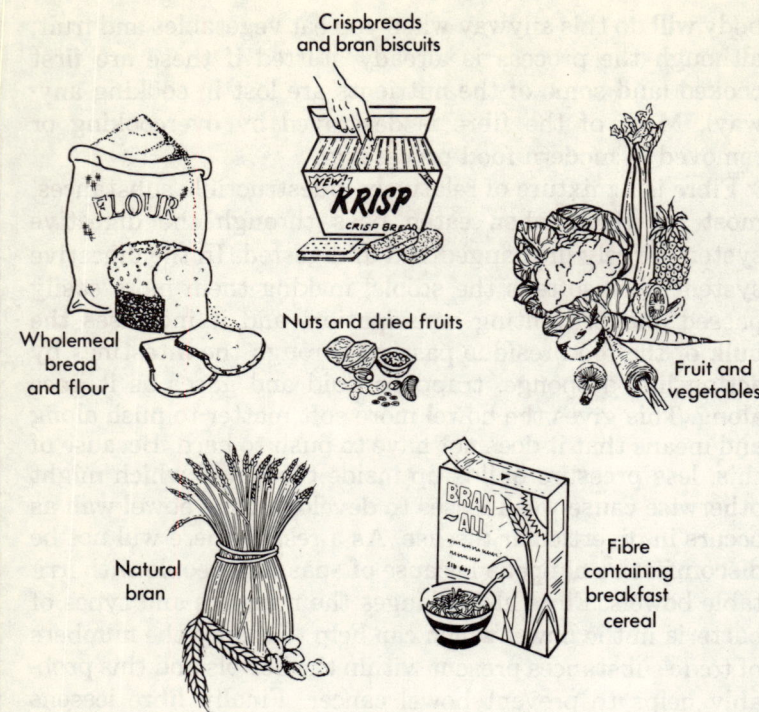

Crispbreads and bran biscuits

Wholemeal bread and flour

Nuts and dried fruits

Fruit and vegetables

Natural bran

Fibre containing breakfast cereal

Fig. 7 The various types of food that have a high fibre content.

flaky raw bran is much better than the fine, powdery variety. However the fine bran settles more, so spoonful for spoonful it is probably just as effective. Fine bran is also more palatable but is more likely to be fattening and many of the bran cereals contain large amounts of sugar and tend to encourage putting on weight. Bran is least conspicuous if mixed with breakfast cereal or porridge, thick soups and sauces, stewed fruit and rice. The amount of bran needed varies greatly from person to person and can only be found out by starting with, for example, one heaped dessert-spoonful daily and gradually increasing it until you can pass a soft, formed stool without undue effort. Bran can be bought from most health food shops. If you really cannot take bran or fibre in any other way your doctor may be able to help you find a way around it. Don't forget, bran may temporarily upset the bowels but you should continue it uninterrupted and things will normally settle back down again. It usually begins to have an effect over a matter of a few days, but may not have its full benefit for perhaps as long as 2–3 months. Have heart though! The problem of fibre-lacking diets has been recognised for some considerable time and at the turn of the last century in Germany, the use of bread made with wood-shavings was advocated to increase the bulk of the motions!

How do I know if I'm eating enough roughage?

Simple, if your diet contains enough fibre, your stools will be soft yet well formed and can be easily passed without great effort. This really does apply to most people and if it doesn't to you then you should probably see your doctor about it.

Many people find that when they start taking in fibre — containing foods the bowel may be upset for a short while and they also notice a great deal of wind and bloating. Do not worry about this and do not stop the fibre foods; it will settle down after a few days. It this continues to bother you, it is probably because you have been over enthusiastic and are now eating too much roughage. Try reducing it a little until your bowels are just right. There is no advantage in eating too much roughage and it could be harmful as well.

What shouldn't I eat?

If I've got Crohn's disease? There are no specific do's and don'ts, but if you have had a lot of small intestine removed or diseased you may find you get less diarrhoea by cutting down on the amount of fat you eat each day. If the bowel is very narrowed in places and you get griping pains, chew your food well, especially vegetables and fruit, and make sure you have a good set of teeth! Fibre in the diet often helps to control bowel symptoms and may have some long-lasting benefits.

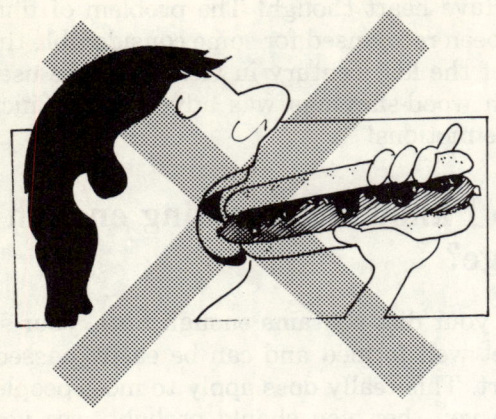

If I've got colitis? Some people find their symptoms are better if they don't have any milk products (cheese, butter, cream, yoghourt). You will only know by trying and this will do you no harm and may mean that you will be able to come off some of your tablets eventually — but only if your doctor tells you to! But don't forget you must not have any milk or anything derived from milk. If it is going to work you should know about it within two or three weeks. Roughage in the diet may help to control the bowels, but it is not known to have any other influence on the disease and will not in anyway be harmful.

If I have an ileostomy? There is nothing that you shouldn't eat and do not worry if you occasionally see unchanged food in the bag. You may find it helpful to cut down on fibre-containing foods, nuts, raw fruits, onions, cabbage and uncooked vegetables, since these can affect odour and wind production. If you suffer from these problems it is best to experiment to find out which foods suit you. You may also find that the time of day you eat can affect the working of your ileostomy.

If I've got coeliac disease? The main aim is, of course, a diet entirely free of gluten. Gluten is present in wheat, rye, barley and oats. Rice, corn and soya bean products are safe. Avoiding wheat in the diet is easier said than done. Flour is added to many foods apart from the obvious, bread, biscuits, cakes, cereals and pasta, and is present in many tinned soups and meats, sauces, gravy mixes, ice-cream, chocolates, most ready-made frozen meals, salad dressings and bed-time drinks. Alcoholic drinks are not usually a problem but it is best to avoid "real" ales and homebrew especially those with sediment in the bottom of the glass. This formidable list is made a little easier by the fact that gluten-free bread and flour can be prescribed. Fortunately, the Coeliac Society keeps up-to-date information on availability of these products and encourages information swapping.

Should I try an exclusion diet?

It is very fashionable nowadays to incriminate food as causing a number of problems, such as asthma, migraine and eczema, as well as multitudinous other disorders. Proof that such diets are beneficial is very hard to come by but, of course, if you believe your diet may be causing you problems it is reasonable to try excluding various items. Do not try this without medical help though, it can be dangerous. It can also be helpful for you to do this in conjunction with a dietitian.

5. HAVE I GOT PILES?

What are piles?

These are also called haemorrhoids and are swollen portions of the delicate lining tissue of the back passage, found near the opening or anus. Although these are extremely common, nobody knows precisely what causes them. Without doubt some people inherit the tendency to develop them. It is known what tends to make them give trouble though and, most commonly, that is straining at stool because of constipation or long-standing diarrhoea. They are also often especially troublesome during or immediately after pregnancy.

When under pressure, the piles and surrounding tissue become very swollen and may protrude out of the back passage (prolapse) and bleed. Constant irritation of this swollen tissue causes inflammation and another common symptom, itching.

How do I know if I've got piles?

Piles commonly bleed and the blood is always bright red — the same colour as if you have just cut your finger. Bleeding usually occurs just after the bowels have been open and may be a little, seen as streaking on the toilet paper, or a gush of

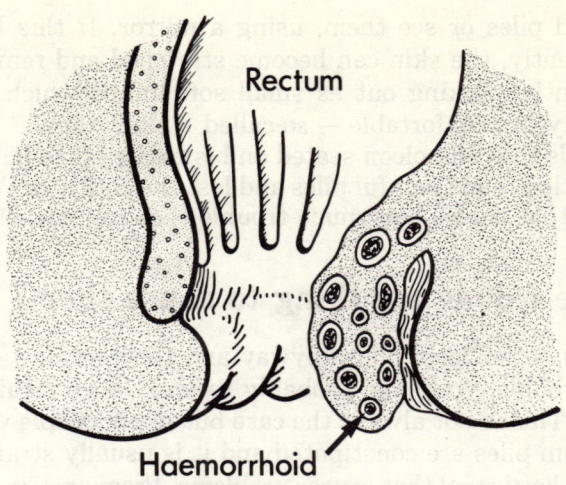

Rectum

Haemorrhoid

Fig. 8 A diagram of how a pile (haemorrhoid) forms. This is an imaginary 'slice' through the back passage (rectum). The pile is a swollen portion of the bowel lining which may stretch down through the back passage opening (the anus).

bright red blood coming away by itself and splattering the toilet pan.

Piles also cause pain or discomfort. This is most commonly, local irritation and itching (called pruritus ani). Piles are amongst the commonest causes of itching around the back passage but this may also be due to sensitivity or infection of the skin surrounding it. The flow of blood through the piles may become blocked off and cause thrombosis of the haemorrhoids. They can also protrude out of the back passage and not slide back in again (and get stuck or 'strangulate'). Either of these problems can cause intense pain in or immediately around the back passage.

Piles can protrude or prolapse through the back passage and normally do so when the bowels are opened. They usually settle back again into the back passage when there is no further straining. On occasions when they remain stuck down they can become very congested and cause discomfort and irritation, and it is sometimes possible to feel the congested piles or see them, using a mirror. If this happens frequently, the skin can become stretched and remain permanently sticking out as small soft lumps which are not usually uncomfortable — so-called "skin tags". History records that Napoleon seated on his battle horse paid much attention to his painful piles and lost the Battle of Waterloo — so that shows how much trouble they can cause!

Have I done anything to cause them?

If you suffer from piles anyway and they are now causing you trouble, you have probably recently been straining at stool. This is not always the case but many people who suffer from piles are constipated and it is usually straining to pass a hard stool that causes problems. Pregnancy is another common situation in which haemorrhoids are troublesome. Obviously there is not a great deal one can do if you are pregnant, apart from avoiding the additional strain of constipation and attention to your diet is the best way of doing that.

Many people believe that sitting on hot radiators as a child causes piles. Now, that is pretty hard to disprove, but there is no proof that this relatively common pre-occupation of school children causes piles later in life!

Will I always suffer?

If you have had piles in the past, then the answer is yes, you probably will, intermittently. Most sufferers from piles have been troubled on occasions since adolescence. Nobody knows why piles usually start then, but once a sufferer you will probably have some symptoms off and on throughout your life. However, in most people they are a minor inconvenience, if at all, and only a small number require treatment for them. If you are a woman and become pregnant, your piles will almost certainly get worse. Anybody who strains at stool and suffers from piles may find that they start causing trouble again, for a while.

Can I do anything to make them better?

The best way is to prevent them causing you any trouble. This is most effectively done by avoiding straining at stool. The most successful way of doing this is to ensure that the bowels are opened regularly without attempting to strain, by means of eating an appropriate diet which enables you to pass a soft, well formed motion. This is most easily done by eating fibre or roughage in the diet (NOT liquid paraffin!) and, if it is properly done, works in most people. If it doesn't for you, you are either not doing it correctly or there is something else wrong and either way you should see your doctor, because only he or she can tell you which is the case. Don't forget it is you and only you that controls if you strain to pass a motion. One way to prevent trouble that has been suggested in the past is to fit a spring-loaded time switch on the lavatory door that ensures no one sits there for more than 2 minutes! Regular baths and good personal hygiene are also important to relieve the symptoms of piles.

Since piles are so common, a great number of creams and other preparations are available from chemists for self medication. Most of them contain local anaesthetics to numb the area causing the discomfort and to relieve pain or itching. Many are also made with either soft paraffin or other components to soften the skin and help relieve inflammation and irritation and some even contain steroids to reduce inflammation. A great many of these are obviously extremely effective, as judged by the amount of advertising accompanying them and apparent commercial success. In moderation most are also safe, although if used regularly some can soften the skin too much so that infection starts. The only problem with self-medication is really whether you have piles in the first place or not. Although not many other conditions cause the combination of symptoms described, on occasions other problems can occur in this region of the body which may require alternative methods of treatment and only your doctor can tell you one way or the other. As a general rule, since it is rather difficult if not impossible and perhaps unpleasant to examine yourself, if you have symptoms of piles it is reasonable, if you are otherwise fit and healthy and have no other disturbances, to try simple forms of treatment yourself such as diet, avoiding straining and perhaps also self-medication with creams from the chemist. However, if you have any doubts, especially because you have noticed other problems, perhaps bowel disturbance, passing blood *mixed in* with the motions, passing slime with the motions, a general feeling of being unwell, weight loss, abdominal pains, if the symptoms do not rapidly settle, or if you are simply worried about new symptoms, the best solution is to see your doctor to be re-assured and advised of the most appropriate treatment. Passing blood from the back passage is something that should always be investigated before attributing the bleeding to piles.

Could I have something else apart from piles?

Yes, indeed you could. Haemorrhoids may be one of the commonest causes of trouble around the back passage but it is by no means the only one.

One of the most frequent conditions to be confused with piles is an *anal fissure*, which is a tear or fine ulcer in the delicate lining of the back passage. This is usually extremely painful, often likened to a red hot needle. It occurs usually during or soon after opening the bowels and the pain can often be prolonged and then feels like a dull aching sensation. Sometimes a period of constipation or diarrhoea brings on the symptoms but it can just come on unexpectedly, although it is probably usually due to straining. Once again, this condition very commonly occurs after a recent pregnancy. A fissure most commonly causes pain, bleeding — usually a streak of bright red blood on the toilet paper, itching, feeling a small lump on the edge of the back passage or discharge from the back passage.

These are best treated in a similar way to piles, by avoiding constipation and straining and, if necessary, applying special creams locally, regular baths and good personal hygiene. Most will heal up by themselves but if they persistently cause trouble it may be necessary to stretch the back passage under anaesthetic in hospital to relieve the muscle spasm that occurs in this condition, or perform an operation to cut the muscles.

Sometimes, due to weakness of the muscles which support the back passage, this can sink downwards and prolapse in a similar manner to the way the womb can prolapse in women. Anyone who suffers from *rectal prolapse* can be conscious of "something coming down" when the bowels are opening and may occasionally have to actually push this part of the rectum back up again afterwards. This particular problem usually requires specialist diagnosis and treatment and this is most commonly carried out in hospital.

A number of other conditions can occur around the back passage and give rise to symptoms similar to all of those previously described. Skin diseases can cause itching and treatment of the actual skin disease is usually important to relieve this symptom. In children itching may be caused by worms. Abscesses can form around the back passage and cause intense throbbing pain and usually require an operation to relieve the discomfort. Leaks (discharging sinuses) from the bowel may also occur in this region and require medical attention. Although these can occur for no obvious reason, it is important to make sure that there is no underlying bowel disease. One type of sinus that can discharge, occurs in the cleft between the buttocks at the base of the spine. This has nothing to do with the bowels but it can often be confused with other problems around the back passage. This is called a *pilonidal sinus* and is probably caused by hair, irritating and breaking down the skin. This leads to a track developing under the skin and usually requires medical attention to settle it sooner or later.

Cancers and benign (non-malignant) growths can occur in or around the back passage and may cause bleeding and discharge with bowel motions. Inflammation of the lining of the back passage can cause similar problems (proctitis). Most frequently bleeding occurs with the blood mixed in the bowel motions and sometimes also a constant feeling of wanting to open the bowels (tenesmus). The only possible way to identify these problems, to avoid confusion with piles, is by consulting a doctor. As a general rule, any cause of bleeding or discharge from the back passage must arouse suspicion and the only way to be certain that it is not due to anything serious is to see a doctor.

Proctalgia fugax is a strange name for a fairly common complaint. In this condition, the affected person suddenly experiences a severe sharp pain in the region of the back passage. It lasts for a few seconds or minutes and disappears as mysteriously as it came. It can occur at any time but is usually in the day and often soon after a bowel movement. It is believed to be caused by spasm in the muscles around the back passage. Women appear to be affected more frequently than men and these people often have symptoms of an irritable bowel as well.

Do piles mean that I've got anything else?

Piles can sometimes be due to some other disorder but in the vast majority of cases they occur in perfectly fit and healthy people. If you read medical books in the library most will contain references to underlying diseases that cause piles. This may very occasionally occur, but piles are so common that the number of people who will have any other cause for haemorrhoids is very small indeed. Looking at it another way, the chance that your piles are due to any other disease is so small as to not be worth even considering. The important thing to be certain about is that the troubles you have are actually due to piles and not to anything else. The only way to be absolutely certain is to be fully medically examined.

What can be done about my piles?

Two hundred years ago it was believed that bleeding from piles was good for you and leeches were sometimes applied to encourage this! Our thinking has now changed and we try to stop bleeding and other symptoms.

In the first place your doctor will probably advise you to follow simple remedies, avoiding straining and constipation. Local creams may be prescribed to reduce the amount of swelling and inflammation of the surrounding tissues and take away your discomfort. If this is unsuccessful and you continue to have troubles or your doctor wants you checked over to rule out other diseases, you may need to go to hospital. Most patients attending hospital for piles are simply examined at the clinic and this is all that is necessary to exclude any other problems. At the same time, the piles may also be treated by injection, which is not nearly so painful as it may sound! An anaesthetic is not usually needed and a special solution is injected around the swelling causing the piles, so that scarring results and the haemorrhoids later shrivel away. Most haemorrhoid sufferers respond to this form of treatment, but an operation may be necessary for those who do not. This usually requires stretching of the back passage under an anaesthetic (a procedure first devised by the Ancient Greeks!) and removal of the haemorrhoids, either by tying them off or surgically removing them.

These forms of treatment are usually very effective in relieving most sufferers but careful attention to diet and avoidance of straining at stool are important to prevent recurrences.

6. WHAT SHOULD I DO ABOUT MY BOWELS?

Do I need to see my doctor about my bowels?

Only if you think that there is something wrong. The most important problems that are likely to be due to a disease of the bowel is a *change* in your bowel habit from what has previously been *normal for you*. If you have noticed that you have become constipated and are passing smaller quantities of stool less frequently or have diarrhoea, passing liquid or poorly formed loose stools more frequently than usual, this is important. Everybody experiences some sort of bowel upset every now and again and it is awfully difficult to say precisely how long you should put up with bowel disturbance before seeing your doctor. A general rule would be that if a marked change occurs in the bowels and persists for more than 2–3 weeks or it is having a noticeable effect on your life — you're always having to rush to the toilet or you have to sit there for half an hour straining away to pass anything at all, then you need to see your doctor. Similarly if you are genuinely worried about your bowels even if there has been no change, but you think your bowels behave differently from everybody else's, the only way to be sure that you are alright is to see your doctor.

The other important clues that you may have a disease of

the bowel are many. The most suggestive are tummy ache or abdominal pain, vomiting and change or disturbance of the bowel, passing blood or slime with the motions, leaking of motions uncontrollably from the back passage and soiling of your clothes, unexplained loss of weight, or lack of energy and no longer feeling well (general malaise and lethargy) together with disturbance of the bowels.

Increase in the size of your tummy (as long as you are not getting fatter — and you can tell this by the "pinch" test!), wind and rumbling of the tummy, may also be caused by bowel disease. Only your doctor can put your mind at rest.

Do bowels tell you about your general health?

Sometimes. There is little truth in the belief that forcing your bowels to open makes you fitter and healthier than you would otherwise be. However, if you are generally ill and run down this may cause bowel upsets. If you are not eating regularly or you are vomiting and there is nothing going in to you, there is obviously less than normal to come out of you! If you are depressed this may affect your life style, as may stress and this can cause bowel disturbance. Some generalised diseases, especially those affecting the thyroid gland, can upset the bowels and drugs taken for other illnesses (antibiotics commonly cause mild diarrhoea) may also affect the bowels. Normally you know that you have something wrong with your general health before the bowels become upset. It is fairly unusual for bowel disturbance by itself to cause some hidden disease elsewhere to come to light.

Can anybody else catch bowel trouble from me?

It is possible depending on what causes your bowel disease.

65

If it is infection, and gastroenteritis is the commonest type of gut infection, you almost certainly caught it from somewhere and could pass it on to others. You probably won't actually know how you caught it, so it is better to play safe. While you are ill, try to avoid handling food, cooking utensils, cutlery or crockery intended for others and wash your hands well especially after going to the toilet. Stay away from young babies and old people if possible. Apart from infections, the only other way you could pass on bowel trouble to someone else is by your children inheriting a tendency towards these diseases — they cannot catch them directly. Coeliac disease, Crohn's disease and ulcerative colitis tend to run in families although the risk is not great. Nobody knows how these diseases are inherited so it is impossible to predict which children, if any, could develop them. People are *not* usually advised to avoid having families because of the risk of passing on bowel diseases.

Are bowel disorders serious?

Some are. Occasionally bowel diseases can be life-threatening but more usually they are simply a nuisance. It is far less likely that a bowel disease which is known about and for which you are being treated will pose any threat to your life, than one from which you suffer and have either ignored the symptoms or have been too frightened to go and see your doctor about.

I don't like to talk about my bowels: will I have to?

Yes, I am afraid you will. The problems caused by bowel diseases are the symptoms you have noticed, that have taken you to the doctor. These are the clues and your doctor will have a good idea by talking to you whether you are likely to have a bowel disease, any other disorder or nothing at all wrong with you.

Will my doctor need to examine me?

It is quite likely unless you have a most unusual doctor with X-ray eyes! However, when your doctor has spoken to you it may be very apparent that there is nothing to worry about but even so your doctor may prefer to check, to be absolutely sure. On the other hand, your doctor may be able to tell as soon as you walk through the door what the matter with you is and be able to take action without asking you to take off your clothes.

I won't have to go to hospital, will I?

It really depends on what your doctor thinks when he or she sees you. You must remember that the intestines lie very deep within your tummy and only fairly obvious problems are going to show on the surface. If your doctor is worried about you or just wants to be absolutely certain that there is nothing wrong, you may be advised to have some further tests. In that case you will almost certainly have to go to hospital, perhaps just to have a test or even see a specialist.

If you do go to see a specialist you will have to tell your story again and almost certainly be fully examined. The specialist will not want to put you through any tests unless absolutely convinced there is a need for them. It is likely that when you are seen at the hospital clinic you will have some blood tests, unless your own doctor has already done these. Blood tests commonly become abnormal at an early stage in many illnesses and often are useful as a guide to whether any disease is present.

Can't my doctors just treat me?

Well I suppose he or she could but the question is with what and for what? Most of the medicines used for bowel diseases themselves, rather than just for the symptoms caused by these diseases, are very specific for each particular disease and will not work in others. Furthermore, constipation and diarrhoea may just be the signal that you have an underlying disease, so it's far better to treat the disease upsetting the bowel, rather than the problem it causes. Would you treat a leaking tap by permanently turning off the stopcock? Isn't it better just to change the washer?

The main reason for wanting to find out if you have an underlying bowel disease is that for many, early treatment makes a lot of difference to what happens in the long run.

What tests will need to be done?

X-rays

X-rays are often one of the first kind of tests that are needed. For most special X-rays the bowel has to be 'prepared' so that it is as clean as possible and can be carefully examined. The X-ray is normally arranged with you for a convenient time and you are given instructions as to whether you can eat or drink beforehand and if any special laxative medicines are necessary to help evacuate the bowel.

Probably the most commonly performed test of the digestive system is a barium X-ray. Barium is a white, thick liquid that shows up on X-ray. It is used to examine the gut by swallowing the barium and waiting until it enters the stomach — a barium meal. After some time the barium enters the small intestine and this can be examined — a barium follow-through. It takes several hours for the barium liquid to pass all the way through the small intestine and by the time it reaches the large intestine it is so mixed with food material that this region cannot be properly inspected. Therefore, to examine the large intestine, barium is inserted through the back passage or rectum by means of a tube (barium enema) and then allowed to flow back around the large intestine (colon). Sometimes in order to improve the quality of the examination, air is also pumped into the large bowel. These tests are usually performed in the X-ray department, with the patient lying on a couch. Pictures are taken as a permanent record, but progress can usually be followed on a television screen. The patient is tilted into a number of different positions so that all the parts of the digestive system can be carefully examined. Other kinds of X-rays may be needed as well.

Endoscopic tests

Endoscopic tests are also commonly used. This procedure simply involves looking inside a person. The most simple method is performed in a clinic or outpatients department when a short, rigid tube is inserted into the back passage (rectum) and the lining illuminated by shining a light down the tube and examined through a 'close-up' lens (sigmoidoscopy). This is a very important and simple test and not too unpleasant. It is a very effective way of examining the bowel lining for inflammation and checking for gut cancers — since most form within the area that can be inspected by this instrument. It also allows samples of tissues (biopsies) to be removed internally with forceps for microscopic examination, to confirm inflammation, cancer or a non-cancerous growth.

An examination may also be needed with a fibreoptic instrument. Fibreoptic are a technique where a powerful light beam can be shone down a bundle of fine glass fibres and an image illuminated at the far end, can be transmitted back to be seen by the operator. The great advantage of this method is that it is possible to see around corners and the instrument can therefore be guided throughout the intestine with all the bends and kinks that this has. A general anaesthetic is seldom required except in children and the instruments are easily passed into the intestines through the rectum — a colonoscopy, after an injection into a vein to make the patient a little drowsy and reduce any discomfort. Once again, for most of these procedures to be successful, the bowel must be cleaned out beforehand.

In people who have been bleeding from the intestines it is often possible using these instruments to find out exactly where the blood is coming from and in some cases stop further bleeding by direct heat coagulation of the blood vessels. Similarly, polyps (small, non-cancerous growths) in the colon can also often be removed with this kind of instrument without a full operation being necessary.

Sometimes, a similar type of instrument is introduced into the abdominal cavity through a small cut in the abdominal wall usually under some form of anaesthetic. This is called a laparoscopy. All of the organs within the abdomen can then be inspected this way without a full exploratory operation (laparotomy) being necessary.

Using all of these methods, tissue fragments can be removed from many areas of the digestive tract (biopsies). The fragments are examined microscopically and the appearances are often an invaluable aid to diagnosis of a number of different conditions. It is particularly important in coeliac disease to remove a portion of small bowel lining to demonstrate the characteristic abnormalities. This is usually carried out using a tube swallowed through the mouth (jejunal biopsy). It is also often extremely helpful to remove a core of liver tissue for diagnosis (liver biopsy). This is usually performed by introducing a fine needle into the liver through the right side, under local anaesthetic and sucking in a small portion of liver tissue. Although this only gives information about the liver it is sometimes necessary to know about this in people with certain bowel diseases.

Motility tests

The functions of the gut can also be measured. The movements in the large intestine (colon) can be assessed by a *motility test*. In this examination, a fine tube is passed through the back passage into the bowel. One end is connected to a measuring gauge and the movements of the bowel recorded. The rate of absorption of foods, glucose and xylose (sugars) from the gut, into the bloodstream can also be measured and the failure to absorb fats assessed by collection of stool samples and the subsequent measurement in these of fat content.

What will my doctor treat me with?

Anti-diarrhoeals (Lomotil, Imodium, Codeine Phosphate, Kaolin)

These compounds act on the bowel by damping down over-active movements of intestine. Some are derived from opiates (morphine) which diminish bowel movement, but have no serious addictive side effects (codeine). Kaolin (a clay) may also be used to add a solidifying effect to loose stools.

Laxatives

These act in a number of different ways. Some, by adding bulk to the motions, sugars (such as Lactulose or Sorbitol) and fibre (Normacol, Fybogel, Fybranta, Proctofibe). Others stimulate and irritate the bowel (Senokot), and glycerol (or paraffin) loosens and lubricates the faeces. Long-term use of laxatives can damage the bowel and there is no place for regular laxatives except under careful medical supervision. In the past poisons such as strychnine and mercury were used for a laxative effect. Modern generation aperients may not be overtly poisonous agents but are not much better than poisons in many respects! There is nothing to commend the practice of giving regular doses of laxatives to normal people and the use of castor oil in children in particular is to be strongly discouraged.

Enemas are also sometimes used, the volume instilled stimulates the bowel to empty. Suppositories are also effective and contain drugs which either stimulate the bowel or lubricate the faeces. These methods of treatment have been used for centuries. Enemas were in common use amongst the ancient Egyptians. In fact they ascribed the discovery of enemas to the bird known as the Ibis. They apparently believed that this creature washed the inside of its body by introducing water with its beak into the intestines! Hippocrates (460 BC) the so-called 'father of medicine' thought that enemas were preferable to the use of purgatives except in especially strong people! He also recommended the use of cylindrical suppositories of honey smeared with ox-bile as a still milder form of treatment!

Treatment around the anus

A number of compounds (e.g. Anusol, Proctofoam) are used in the treatment of uncomfortable conditions around the anus. Most contain local anaesthetic to relieve discomfort and a small dose of anti-inflammatory drugs (commonly steroids) to reduce swelling and inflammation.

Antispasmodics

These drugs relieve spasm in the bowel, and are usually propantheline (Probanthine), mebeverine (Colofac), dicyclomine (Merbentyl) or peppermint oil capsules (Colpermin). Some can cause side effects, in particular dryness of the mouth and blurring of vision, but most do not.

Corticosteriods (prednisone or prednisolone)

These are used mainly to treat inflammatory bowel conditions. They may be used as a tablet, by injection or as an enema to treat inflammation of the intestine particularly due to Crohn's disease or ulcerative colitis. Their use in large doses may be associated with a number of side effects and because of this, whenever possible, direct application to the inflamed bowel by enemas is used. The commonest side effects caused by prednisone or prednisolone are rounding of the face, bruising, an increase in appetite, mood changes, thinning of the bones, muscles and skin, a general 'muzziness' around the head and eyes, temporary high blood pressure and occasionally a temporary diabetes. Other drugs which reduce inflammation, particularly azathioprine (Imuran) may also occasionally be used in inflammatory bowel diseases (Crohn's disease or ulcerative colitis).

Sulphasalazine (Salazopyrin)

This is a drug used in the treatment of ulcerative colitis and Crohn's disease. It is a combination of a sulphonamide (a type of antibiotic) and a derivative of aspirin. However, it does not act in the same manner as the component drugs, but, when given by mouth or enema is split in the large bowel by bacteria to produce a local anti-inflammatory effect. It is very effective in keeping the inflammatory damage controlled and preventing recurrence of symptoms when taken on a long-term basis. It can cause nausea or vomiting, skin rashes or anaemia and the effects may be abolished by a reduction in dose or by using sugar-coated tablets. It may also be used as an enema to give a topical effect. It frequently causes the urine to turn darker and sometimes a deep orange colour but this is nothing to worry about — although you should let your doctor know about it if this happens.

Antibiotics (Metronidazole — Flagyl, Neomycin)

May be used to treat infections of the intestines or during bowel operations. They may be used to have a local effect in the gut by giving a type that is not absorbed into the body — such as Neomycin. Alternatively a variety that enters the bloodstream and has a generalised effect throughout the body may be used. Some antibiotics are so effective at killing bacteria within the gut that they may lead to overgrowth of fungi — particularly in the mouth to give 'thrush'. Alternatively antibiotics themselves may cause diarrhoea. Alcoholic drinks should not be taken if you are on a course of metronidazole as this combination causes unpleasant effects.

What kinds of operation are done on the bowel?

Many types of intestinal operations are performed, depending upon the problem and which part of the gut is affected.

The technical names for operations are often bewildering. In general terms removal of an organ is described by the anatomical name followed by *-ectomy,* e.g. colectomy (removal of the colon), appendicectomy (removal of the appendix). Alternatively making a permanent opening in an organ is described by the term *-ostomy,* e.g. ileostomy (making a hole in the ileum).

Many operations are carried out on the digestive system and most are described by such terms. Usually the affected part is removed and the remaining intestines sewn back together again. Since the intestines are so large, quite long lengths can be removed without causing any obvious ill-effects. If it is not possible to join the remaining parts of the gut together it may be necessary to make the intestine empty onto the surface of the tummy — an ileostomy or colostomy.

The faecal contents then pass into a bag which is emptied periodically. This might be thought to be unpleasant and difficult to manage because of the accumulation of wind within the bag, odour and irritation of the surrounding skin. However, many appliances are available to overcome these problems and nearly all patients who require this surgery learn to adapt very well. However, the initial problems are often very trying and those who are attempting to cope may require sympathy and understanding, particularly in the early days. This type of surgery is, however, compatible with a perfectly normal life afterwards and there is even some evidence to suggest that people who have undergone these operations actually lead fuller lives than before!

What should I know if I have an ileostomy or colostomy?

An *-ostomy* means that the bowel ends and opens as a spout (or stoma) on to the abdominal wall instead of into the back passage or another part of the bowel. If it is the small bowel that opens, this is called an ileostomy; if it is the large bowel, a colostomy.

In general, the problems for most people with any opening on to the tummy wall are similar. If the opening is an ileostomy, the motion emptying out is liquid, may be smelly, irritant and full of gas. If any of the large intestine remains and a colostomy is made, some of these problems should be lessened. With a colostomy it is often possible to learn the colostomy's 'habit' or the times it normally functions and this can be controlled by manipulating the diet and the times of meals. This is not usually so for an ileostomy, however, because the discharge comes from higher up in the digestive system where water and digestive secretions have not yet been fully removed and it is considerably more liquid in consistency. An ileostomy is most active after meals but its activity is highly irregular and it cannot be satisfactorily controlled. Because of this, people with ileostomies must wear a fitted pouch or appliance at all times to collect the liquid discharge and to protect their skin from the irritating effects of the digestive juices which are not found in normal stools.

For an ileostomy, two main types of appliance are available. In one, the bag can be washed and used repeatedly and it is usually attached to the tummy wall by a separate flange that adheres to the skin around the stoma. In the other, the bag and flange are combined in a single device which is usually disposable. Most bags used are those made by Hollister, Chiron & Downs (the Readyfit). Although many of these appliances adhere to the skin, most people wearing them, fearing leakage, use some additional form of support, such as a belt, and use Karaya gum to seal the appliance at the skin to prevent leakage. Most need to change their appliance every few days, but some people can manage up to a week. The bags, of course, need emptying in between this.

There is no reason why someone with an ileostomy cannot live an entirely normal life. Obviously it helps if the stoma works well for you, but an awful lot depends on your attitude to the stoma. If you want to live normally with it (and, if you are a determined person, you will), it is possible to work and take holidays reasonably normally, swim and bathe, enjoy recreational pursuits and sex, but obviously you will first have to learn some of the various 'tricks' that will help you to do these things.

There are also, of course, some problems that can occur with ileostomies. Soreness of the surrounding skin is common and may be due to irritation by bowel contents or an allergic reaction to the materials used with the appliance, especially skin adhesives. Stomahesive is a protective material that is used to help prevent this and Karaya gum discs and barrier creams are also available to prevent direct contact of irritants with the skin. Some bags are made of rubber and this can commonly cause irritation. Most people prefer either an opaque bag, or make a cover for their appliance so that they do not see the contents. Other problems which cause worries are wind forming in the bag, especially at night, and odour, particularly if the bag needs emptying in public toilets. Although charcoal filters and deodorants are available, none is terribly satisfactory. If you suffer with these difficulties, in the first instance it is usually worth making alterations to your diet to avoid wind and odour forming foods. Many find that roughage-containing foods cause wind, and onions, beans, nuts, beer and highly spiced food, particularly curries, are notorious! Sometimes eating the main meal earlier in the day helps the problem of wind forming during the night. Some people find eating chlorophyll or charcoal biscuits help.

What if I have to have a digestive operation?

If you do it will be necessary for the intestines to be cleared out as for the special tests you had performed. It is very important that this is done meticulously to prevent any problems during the operation. You may also need some other tests to prepare you for the anaesthetic and operation — checks on the heart and lungs. Before the operation you should discuss with the surgeon and anaesthetist *exactly* what is wrong with you and what operation is planned before you sign the form to give your consent. Do *not* be afraid to ask — it is your right to know what is going to happen to *your* body. It may also be helpful for you to know what to expect after the operation.

Any operation on the digestive system can lead to temporary inactivity of the gut. Because of this, a short period of drainage, particularly of the stomach may be needed, by means of a tube passed through the nose or mouth to remove the secretions, until recovery occurs. During these early days after surgery, if the digestive tract cannot be used for drink and food, replacement may need to be given into a vein by an intravenous drip.

After any intestinal operation the bowels may not work normally again for some time. Soon after the operation most people are constipated and when the bowels do work, diarrhoea is very common. Although this usually settles after a while, sometimes it can take a considerable time.

7. WHAT WILL MY DOCTOR DO FOR MY BOWELS?

What can be done about gastroenteritis?

Normally the illness will clear up by itself in a few days to a week. Anybody who has had diarrhoea for more than 10 days or 2 weeks should see their doctor since tests may need to be carried out and treatment started. Gastroenteritis may be confirmed by growth of the infecting organism from the faeces or blood, but this cannot be done satisfactorily in a large number of cases. During the illness, it is best to eat little, but to keep having plenty to drink, particularly drinks that contain sugar (such as Lucozade), and perhaps also with a pinch of salt added, especially in hot climates. Rest is also often beneficial. Anti-diarrhoeal and anti-sickness treatment may be prescribed by the doctor if the symptoms continue. Antibiotics are not often helpful in the actual illness but may be used to treat any infection which has not been spontaneously eliminated from the body. They may be positively harmful in some situations. Antibiotics can cause diarrhoea themselves, or in typhoid (which is still fairly common in this country) they may prevent the body eradicating the infection by itself. Don't forget that the sudden onset of diarrhoea is usually due to infection and is in itself a protective mechanism serving to clear the gut of the organisms causing the illness. On common sense grounds it is arguably better to let the infection run its course as the body will clear the organism by itself in most cases. Since this is of course sometimes unpleasant and inconvenient, there is no reason to think that buying simple medicines such as kaolin from the chemist will do any harm. Probably the best and most effective medicine that your doctor may prescribe is Loperamide or Lomotil which help to diminish the overactivity of the gut and cut down the intestinal secretions caused by the irritation.

How will my doctor know if I have coeliac disease?

It is diagnosed by blood tests showing an anaemia and sometimes a barium X-ray (follow-through examination)

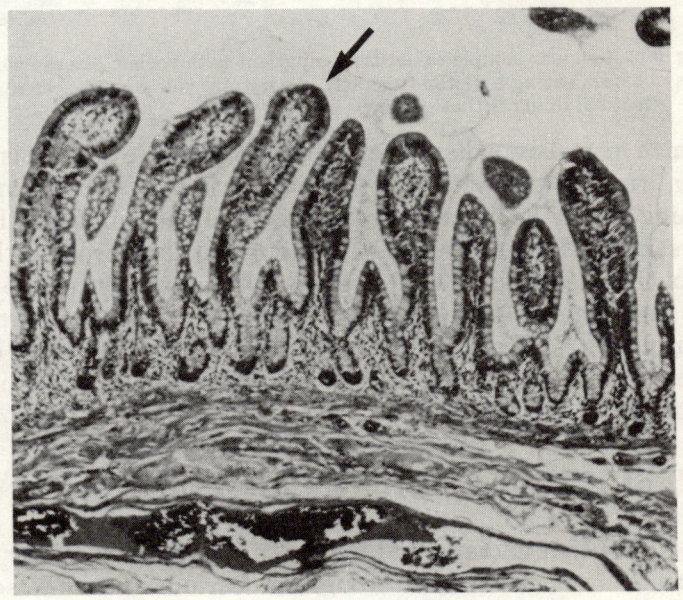

Fig. 9(a) A sample of the intestinal lining enlarged many times under a microscope. The normal 'finger-like' villi (marked with an arrow) can be seen projecting into the hollow inside of the bowel.

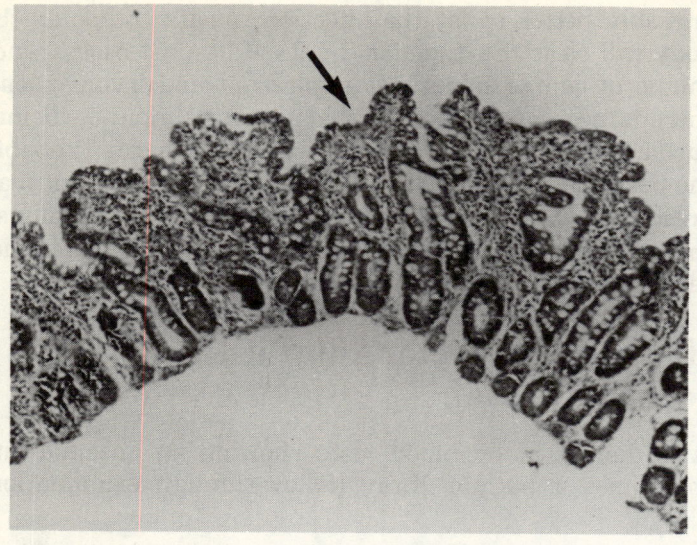

Fig. 9(b) A similar sample taken from a patient with coeliac disease who has not been eating a gluten-free diet. The normal villi are not seen and the intestinal lining is 'flat' (arrow).

which may show a disturbance of digestion. The diagnosis is confirmed by examination of a small section of the intestinal lining under the microscope. This is easily accomplished by passing a fine tube under X-ray guidance through the mouth and down into the upper part of the small intestine (a jejunal biopsy). It is usual for this test to be repeated after a period of treatment on a diet without wheat, rye, oats or barley (i.e. a gluten-free diet) to confirm that the intestinal lining is healing.

What if I've got Crohn's disease?

The condition is diagnosed by X-ray examination (either a barium meal and follow-through, or barium enema — see p. 67) but it may also be necessary to confirm the diagnosis by endoscopic assessment (colonoscopy or gastroscopy) or operation.

Treatment for severe activity of the disease may require admission to hospital and bed rest, together with treatment which includes blood transfusion, nutritious diets, vitamin supplements and anti-inflammatory treatment. This usually means prednisone or prednisolone (corticosteroids) and Salazopyrin (Sulphasalazine) which settle down the inflammation. This disorder is life-long and results in recurrence of symptoms at unpredictable times. These are usually kept under control by anti-inflammatory drugs. However, since the anti-inflammatory drugs in themselves can cause problems, they are used sparingly and only in specific circumstances. If drug treatment alone fails to control the symptoms, surgery may be necessary to remove the affected bowel. This can often be accomplished entirely internally within the abdomen and the remaining bowel subsequently sewn back together again to restore continuity. If it is not possible to do this, it may instead be necessary to create an artificial opening of the bowel onto the abdominal wall either temporarily or permanently (an ileostomy or colostomy). The disease can recur after surgery, often where the bowel has been joined back together again internally. Because of this, surgical treatment is only usually recommended when there is a particular reason to prefer this option to drug treatment. Most patients with Crohn's disease do, however, need at least one operation at some time or other. Surgery is also often required for specific complications of the disease. Some of the reasons are when the bowel becomes very narrowed or it leaks spontaneously through into another loop of bowel or on to the wall of the tummy — a fistula.

Digestion is often affected in Crohn's disease and sufferers may need additional food or vitamin supplements in the long-term to prevent anaemia and thinning of the bones in particular. Although there is no specific curative treatment for Crohn's disease, the vast majority of sufferers learn to control the disease very satisfactorily with careful medical supervision and live entirely normal lives. There is no close association between this disease and cancer.

Could I have colitis?

Ulcerative colitis is diagnosed by barium enema examination and confirmed by examination of the lining of the large bowel through the back passage (rectum) and removal of a piece of tissue for microscopic study (biopsy).

It is treated in a similar manner to Crohn's disease, although patients are more often treated in the long-term with Salazopyrin (Sulphasalazine) since this is very effective

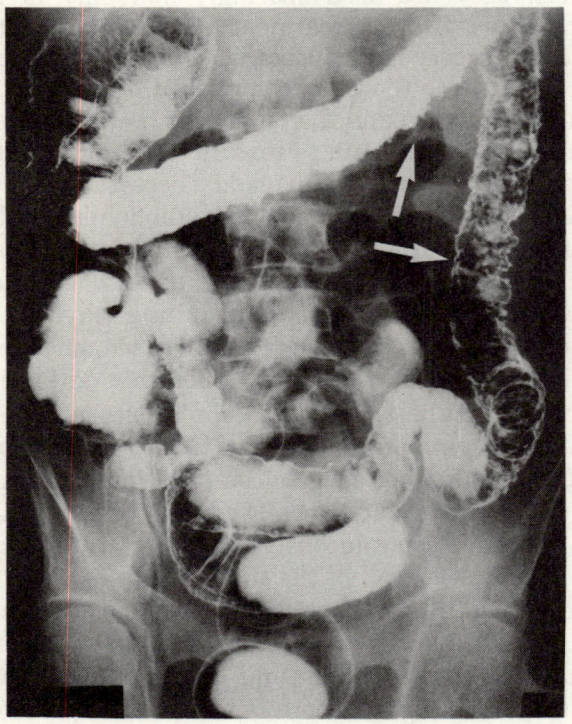

Fig. 10 A barium enema X-ray showing the large bowel in a patient with ulcerative colitis. The edge of the bowel (marked with the arrows) is irregular and 'ragged' because of the ulceration and damage affecting the bowel lining.

in damping down the disease and preventing the recurrences. In order to minimise the amount of prednisolone needed by mouth to settle active disease, this may be given as a suppository or enema directly into the bowel through the back passage or rectum (Predsol, hydrocortisone, Cortenema, Colifoam, etc.). Long-standing extensive disease (colitis) may cause chronic ill health or may after many years lead to bowel cancer. To prevent this, patients who have suffered from the disease for many years, or those whose lives are threatened by severe disease which does not respond to other forms of treatment are often recommended to undergo surgery. This usually involves the removal of the entire large bowel at operation and the creation of an artificial bowel opening on the abdominal wall (ileostomy). Once this is done the disease is cured and cannot recur. If the colon can be left, because of the cancer risks, it may be necessary to check the lining of the bowel periodically by colonoscopy and repeat biopsies. It is possible in many cases to predict if a cancer is likely to develop by these means and to reduce the necessity for operations intended to prevent cancer developing.

Ulcerative colitis and Crohn's disease are the only long-standing conditions commonly occurring in this country that cause inflammation of the colon and are strictly the only types of colitis. This term is, however, often loosely (and incorrectly) applied to a number of other colonic problems.

What will be done if I have appendicitis?

The diagnosis first has to be confirmed at examination by a doctor. Urgent operation is required to prevent the appendix bursting. This is usually performed through a small diagonal incision over the appendix area (the lower right side of the tummy region above the groin), but if there is any doubt about the diagnosis or if difficulties are encountered, a larger incision may be necessary. If performed early, the appendix is simply removed and the opening remaining in the bowel stitched over, recovery normally only taking a few days. However, if peritonitis has occurred as a result of the appendix bursting, recovery may take longer. Sometimes the appendix can slowly leak and lead to an abscess forming. In these circumstances, the infection is usually first settled using antibiotics before operation is performed. Infection and inflammation of the bowel, infections in the urine or vagina spreading to involve the kidneys or ovaries can often mimic appendicitis. Since the diagnosis is occasionally difficult and there is no specific test to confirm appendicitis, it is sometimes safer to remove a normal appendix if appendicitis is suspected, rather than to wait and risk the development of peritonitis, if appendicitis were otherwise missed. Once the appendix is removed, appendicitis cannot recur. A few people suffer from chronic pain which may or may not be due to a 'grumbling' appendix. Whether this entity truly exists is controversial but on occasion operation may be advised and this sometimes resolves the symptoms.

If I have an irritable bowel, can anything be done about it?

Yes of course it can and it is often very easily treated. It is helpful to understand what is going on and very important to make sure that more serious bowel conditions are not causing your problems.

The diagnosis is made, from the very typical story of abdominal discomfort and bowel disturbance often aggravated by stress, in an otherwise well person. Distension giving a 'blown up' feel to the tummy especially towards the end of the day is also common. The abdominal pain can be felt anywhere in the tummy region but is often a lower abdominal nagging discomfort which gets better when the bowels are opened. When these symptoms first start, it is common for more frequent motions (especially in the mornings, soon after getting out of bed, for some strange reason) and looser motions to also occur. Often the symptoms follow an obvious attack of gastroenteritis, commonly those starting on holidays abroad. There is usually

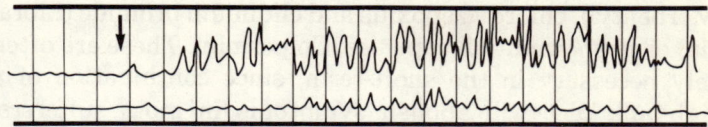

Fig. 11 A recording of the normal movements of the intestine is shown on the left hand side of the arrow. Movements of the bowel are usually indicated by a rise and fall of the line on the tracing and very little is occurring. This recording is taken from a patient with an irritable colon who eats a meal at the point marked by the arrow. Immediately after the meal, the intestinal movements become extremely active and the patient soon has to run to the toilet to open the bowels.

nothing abnormal to find on examination, except for some localised tenderness over the colon and a barium enema examination can show either spasm of the bowel or diverticula or may be entirely normal.

A number of years ago it was customary to advise sufferers to reduce the bulk or residue in the diet. However, it is now apparent that this is usually not the best treatment and it is much more common nowadays to recommend a high fibre or bulk diet. Fibre is contained in foods such as bran, All Bran, Bran Buds, wholewheat and wholemeal bread and biscuits, and uncooked or lightly cooked fresh vegetables. White bread, most ordinary brown breads, doughnuts, pastries, cakes and biscuits, cornflakes and many other cereals are highly processed and the fibre content low and these should be avoided, as should sugar and sweetened foods. It is important to realise that when one starts a high bulk diet, flatulence or wind and increased bowel activity may occur after the first few days. However, when the diet is continued long-term, the bowel motions or faeces will increase in bulk and consistency, become well formed, and tend to float in the lavatory. Other symptoms often subside over a matter of weeks. Bulk forming medicines such as Fybogel, Proctofibe and Fybranta may also help to maintain the bulk in the diet, but they are unnecessary in most patients. Associated bowel spasm may be reduced by the use of anti-spasmodics such as mebeverine (Colofac), dicyclomine (Merbentyl), chlordiazepoxide and clidinium bromide (Libraxin) or peppermint oil capsules (Colpermin). These are often only necessary in the short-term, since continuation of a high-bulk diet will abolish symptoms in most sufferers. Most people on a high bulk diet find that they do not need to avoid other foods, apart from occasional ones that they find tend to aggravate symptoms, such as milk, nuts and baked beans, which may increase wind formation. Abdominal bloating and distension is most commonly due to these conditions, although some anxious people also swallow considerable quantities of air, which adds to the bloated feeling.

Diverticular disease often causes symptoms in the same way as if the bowel was just irritable and is usually treated in a similar manner. Occasionally when the symptoms flare up suddenly and are severe, making the patient ill, further treatment may be needed. Acute diverticular disease usually requires bed-rest, often in hospital, and administration of antibiotics and sometimes intravenous fluids and pain-relieving drugs, until it settles spontaneously. However, on occasions surgery may be necessary. If diverticular disease fails to respond to other forms of treatment, it may also be necessary to resort to surgery to remove the affected portion of bowel at operation, although this is not commonly necessary nowadays.

Can bowel cancer be treated?

Yes, in nearly all cases and usually very successfully. It is one of the few cancers which can often fairly easily be completely cured. Some, but not all, of the factors which cause bowel cancer are also known and if any are found they can often be treated and cancer prevented.

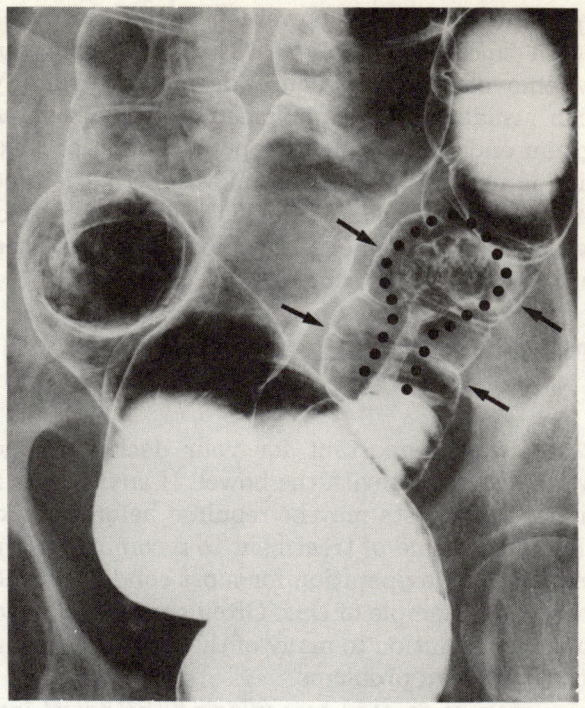

Fig. 12 A barium X-ray of part of the large intestine. A large polyp or protrusion can be seen (outlined by black dots) within the hollow centre of the bowel (shown by arrows). This caused the patient to bleed from the back passage and was removed to prevent the development of cancer.

Diagnosis of intestinal cancer is usually made by examination of the patient, a barium enema X-ray and sometimes colonoscopic examination (see p. 68). Treatment in most cases is by surgery and often the growth and surrounding bowel is easily removed completely and the remaining bowel joined back together internally. Sometimes this may not be possible and a temporary or permanent artificial bowel opening has to be made on the abdominal wall. Drug treatment may also be necessary in addition to, or occasionally instead of, surgery.

Polyps which form in the bowel can sometimes, over many years, turn cancerous. If polyps are known to exist, they are usually removed to prevent cancer developing in later years. This can usually be accomplished nowadays internally through an endoscope (colonoscope) although occasionally operation is necessary. Some families inherit the tendency to develop polyps. If an individual is known to be affected it may be necessary to remove the colon, to prevent the subsequent development of cancer.

Are all bowel troubles treated in the same way?

No. It is always important for your doctor to discover exactly what is wrong with the bowel. If anything is found to be amiss other tests may be required before it is known which is the best kind of treatment to recommend. There is an alternative to an operation for most conditions and hernias are a good example of this. Often surgery provides the best, long-term solution to many of these disorders, but it is not without its own problems.

Hernias may be treated by replacing the bowel into the abdomen and wearing a truss to prevent a recurrence, or by surgical repair of the abdominal wall weakness. It is important to remove any predisposing factors such as obesity or coughing due to excessive smoking, to prevent recurrences.

Other conditions, especially intussusception or volvulus of the bowel, Meckel's diverticulum or appendicitis can occasionally be managed without surgery but most patients require an operation if they have one of these conditions.

APPENDIX

Where else can I turn for help?

There are a number of self-help organisations for patients with various digestive disorders. Most provide information and advice of particular help to people who are newly diagnosed. There are also a great number of local groups serving similar functions and covering defined geographical areas. This is a list of the main national organisations:

National Association for Colitis & Crohn's Disease,
3 Thorpefield Close,
St. Albans, Herts.

The Coeliac Society,
P.O. Box 181,
London NW2 2QY.

The Cystic Fibrosis Research Trust,
5 Blyth Road,
Bromley, Kent. BR1 3RS.

The Colostomy Welfare Group,
38-39 Eccleston Square (2nd floor),
London SW1V 1PB.

The Ileostomy Association of Great Britain & Ireland,
149 Harley Street,
London W.1.

Medic-Alert Foundation,
11/13 Clifton Terrace,
London N4 3JP.
(provides medical identity bracelets and a file on your medical condition for emergencies)

Is there anything I can do to help?

Yes there is. If you suffer from any chronic digestive complaint you may well be able to help others who suffer through the many patient-run, self-help organisations or through your local family doctor or hospital.

You can also help with the provision of information and research into digestive disorders through the British Digestive Foundation. Intestinal diseases are so common and often troublesome that there is considerable scope for a great deal of research. The British Digestive Foundation is one of the newest medical Foundations which have been started to provide support for medical research and information for patients and for the public, particularly in regard to the prevention of illness. This is an organisation run by the public with doctors providing the necessary expert advice, and further information can be obtained from:

The British Digestive Foundation,
7 Chandos Street,
Cavendish Square,
LONDON W1A 2LN.